BEYOND DIFFERENCE

BEYOND DIFFERENCE

AL CONDELUCI, PH.D.

S_L^t

St. Lucie Press
Delray Beach, Florida

Direct all inquiries to:
St. Lucie Press, Inc.
100 E. Linton Blvd., Suite 403B
Delray Beach, Florida, 33483.
Phone: (407) 274-9906
Fax: (407) 274-9927

S_L^t

St. Lucie Press
Delray Beach, Florida

DEDICATION

To Liz

The many years
the love, the tears
the anchor and the seed
the strength to grow
to learn, to know
fulfillment of the need.

Contents

Preface

Preface

The tenor of our world has changed. If you look around, the signs are everywhere. I'm not speaking of the current political and social rhetoric of diversity, multi-culturalism, and inclusion. Indeed, we hear of these things daily in reports from our government, schools, and committees, and many of us embrace these notions.

My reference point for change is found more in the behavior and actions of people and systems. Although it is suspect to generalize, I call you to examine actions and patterns of people and organizations that you know in your life. Certainly, patterns vary, but to me it seems as if our society, and its institutions, are becoming more and more calculating, predictive, specialized, and mechanical.

By institutions, I am referring to the structured actions, formal and informal, of our society. Sociologists (Bellah, et al., 1991) define an institution as:

> a pattern of expected action of individuals or groups enforced by social sanctions, both positive and negative...institutions may be such a simple custom as the confirming handshakes in a social situation...or they may be highly formal institutions such as taxation upon which social services depend. (p. 10)

The notion of institutional change and the mechanistic tenor of its impact is all around us. Our schools, for example, offer an interesting lens for analysis. Although their goal is to prepare a well rounded citizen, they work hard to help students develop technical skills and focus on a standard scale. Some argue that a broad basis of exposure has been diluted and distilled (Bloom, 1987), leading way to a very narrow student, one who is missing in the broader interpretation of the work around them.

Businesses, too, promote workers to become more proficient through uniformity, and often the lure to comply is found in a promotion or raise that keeps the workforce standardized. We have harnessed tools, machines, and more recently, computers and high technology, to enhance our personal and corporate abilities, expand our memories, and allow us an even greater sense of specificity.

As I examine my own field, disability rights and human services, I see this continued quest toward accountability, objectivity, and precision. We strive to enhance policies and procedures to guide our work and there is a premium on predictability. Terms such as *units of service, slots for service, management by objectives,* and *zero based budgets* have become the norm, and anyone associated with human services have felt this mechanization.

To a certain extent, mechanization seems rational and logical and my point in raising this is not to berate technical specialities or the notion of accountability. All organized efforts need a detailed, structured side to them. There would be chaos and dysfunction without an organized format. In fact, it seems that this march to mechanization is a direct response to the importance of organization. The past 20 years in human services, there has been great interest in more succinctly predictable approaches.

This type of organizational influence however, creates an interesting situation. To a large extent, organizations mirror the tenor of the people who comprise them. Often, it is hard to say if organizations influence the individual or that the individual influence the organization. In the *Good Society*, Bellah and associates state:

Institutions are patterns of social activity that give shape to collective and individual experience. An institution is a complex whole that guides and sustains individual identity...

Institutions form individuals by making possible or impossible certain ways of behaving and relating to others. They shape character by assigning responsibility, demanding accountability, and providing the standards in terms of which each person recognizes the excellence of his or her achievements. Each individual's possibilities depend on the opportunities opened up within the institutional contexts to which that person has access... Institutions, then, are essential bearers of ideals and meanings; yet in the real world the embodiment is imperfect. (p. 40)

This assertion that institutions shape character through assigning responsibility, demanding accountability, and providing standards is an important one. If our institutions are becoming more mechanical and robotic, then so will our character.

One organizational theorist, Margaret Wheatley (1992), contends that this trend towards dysfunctional mechanization relates to the fact that most organizations are caught in a Newtonian reality that does not acknowledge current realities. In *Leadership and the New Science*, she states:

It is interesting to note just how Newtonian most organizations are. The machine imagery of the spheres was captured by organizations in an emphasis on structure and parts. Responsibilities have been organized into functions. People have organized into roles. Page after page of organizational charts depict the workings of the machine, the numbers of pieces, what fits where, who the big pieces are... This reduction into parts and the proliferation of separations has characterized not just organizations, but everything in the world during the past three hundred years. Knowledge was broken into disciplines and subjects, engineering became a prized science, and people were fragmented – counseled to use different "parts" of themselves in different settings... A world based on machine images is a world filled with boundaries. In a machine, every piece knows its place. Likewise, in Newtonian organizations, we've drawn boundaries everywhere. We've created roles and accountabilities drawing lines of authority and limits to responsibilities. We have been drawn boundaries around the flow of experience, thus shaping the way we think about the world. (pp. 27-28)

Indeed it seems to me that this structural, predictable side of organizational reality is at runaway proportions. Further, this mechanical domination is not just in human services, but other fields as well. My friend, Karen, a knowledgeable and astute attorney, tells me about trends in her field and the stories sound the same. In her firm, time is highly structured and the value drive in law today is to produce and bill the maximum amount of hours and although Karen holds her own in this flow, she is regularly mocked by colleagues, because she does so much pro bono work and volunteer service in our community.

Karen recently told me a story about a situation in which she sat in judgement, involving a landlord and tenant dispute. The tenant, a single, African-American mother was behind in rent and the landlord was taking action. Karen sat as a legal mediator and as she looked into the eyes of the tenant at the hearing she saw a woman who was dealing with the draw of life, struggling to launch her children, trying to make it work. On the other side was the landlord, owner of multiple properties, wanting to collect his rent.

As she was called to judge the situation, her legal training advanced the letter of the law, the facts of the case and the precision of the matter. In this structured reality, the law is clear, the case is an open and closed one. Pay up or get out.

Yet, in another analysis, one built more from the spirit than the antiseptics of the law, there was much more to this case. Here was a woman, struggling, working hard, probably underpaid and overworked, trying to guide her family, to make it happen. Do these facts alone make her position acceptable or absolve her from paying the rent — of course not. But they should count for something and

Karen works in a world where acknowledgment of the human factors seems to happen less and less.

Another example of mechanization comes from my brother, Dave, a dedicated and committed teacher. He tells me regularly about the growing sterility in his field. He explains how the line has been clearly drawn and teachers can go only so far for risk they may get too close to their students. It seems that each year a new policy that creates even more distance and structure between teachers and students are levied in the school where he taught.

In *Dumbing Us Down*, by John Gatto (1992), the frightening reality of mechanization of school is driven home. As a 25 year veteran of teaching school and recipient of both the New York City and New York State Teacher of the year award, Gatto has come to the conclusion that our formal schooling procedure is ridged, shallow and, in his words, anti-life. He states:

> Ultimately, how we think about social problems depends on our philosophy of human nature: what we think people are, what we think they are capable of, what the purposes of human existence may be, if any. If people are machines then school can only be a way to make those machines more reliable; the logic of machines dictates that parts be uniform and interchangeable, all operations time constrained, predictable, economical. Does this sound like the school you attended, that your children attend?... American education teaches by its methodology that people are machines. Bells ring, circuits open and close, energy flows or is constructed, qualities are reduced to a numbering system, a plan is followed of which the machine parts know nothing. (p. 98)

Clearly, Gatto makes a strong point. Education can become so structured and formalized that most children I know have learned to dislike it. We have taken something as natural as learning and framed it with a mechanical system that has stunted curiosity in an attempt to "order" education.

However, beyond this, is the haunting reality that each generation of students, molded by a system that quantifies, orders, ring bells, separates and sanction difference, then enters our adult world conditioned in a stiff and technical way. These future stewards will not be ready for community diversity and will be roadblocks to an effort attempting to get beyond difference.

I was at a meeting not long ago, where a key topic among the human service administrators present was the necessity to be discreet when called for a reference check. The person leading the discussion said we must be careful not to say too much about a former employee for fear that we might set up a backlash. They recommended that our agencies create a policy where the only facts we offer on a reference check is verification the person worked for us, the dates, and that is all.

Another friend was telling me how their personnel department had reworked personnel policies at his accounting firm to establish a consistent uniformity. It happened that they were taken to task for different standards by an embittered ex-employee. The company was challenged for not being uniform in practice. My friend told me that prior to this action his firm had attempted to respond to the workforce individually. That is, the supervisors tried to factor in unique elements that were inherent to each worker. The embittered employee cried foul and suggested the company's individualist approach was unfair.

Although these observations are anecdotal, they alarm me about the changes happening around us. How is it that mechanization and other narrow social trends have become so rooted that our society is finding it hard to balance for a common good? Bellah and Associates (1985, 1991) suggest that social residue from various junctures of massive impact such as the industrial revolution, development of technology and the shift to computerization have caused major impact. An article that appeared in the Philadelphia Inquier, by Blonston (1992) entitled, *The American Dream*, reported on the changes in communities and made this stark summary:

Americans have become greedy, narrow minded, atomized, individualistic, without a sense of community.

This conclusion, seemingly caused by the effects of the narrowness and mechanization within our society, is a strong indictment, but one few social commentators can argue with. The same Inquirer piece goes on to state:

Money, telecommunications, activist government, individualism, interstate highways, suburbs, the Walmart at the edge of town. They are the talismans of progress, convenience and choice, but they also are the focus that have left so many feeling the loss of close connections.

These notions of uniformity, precision, distance, and structure are becoming more and more of the reality. They have been growing so quickly that they now seem to haunt us and, I believe, to a certain extent, bleed our souls. I think they are creating a robotic, predictable citizen, one who is not only distanced from their neighbor but highly suspicious of people different from the norm. The trend seems to be that people must be all alike, and if not, the agenda is to fix or change people who differ – to fit the uniform.

Another tell-tale sign of the effects of mechanization might be found when looking at the leading cultural indicators in the United States. These cultural indicators have been developed by various national think tanks display some dramatic themes. One interesting review (Bennett, 1994b), for example, displayed five key indicators that are on the rise are:

	1970	1980	1990
Numbers of crimes committed (percentage in millions)	.75	1.3	1.9
Child poverty (percentage of children who are poor)	15%	19%	21%
Teen suicide rate (No. per 100,000 15-24 years old)	6	8	10
Single parent families (percentage of all families with children)	12%	22%	26%
Daily TV viewing (hours of TV viewing per household)	6	6.5	7

Although there can be a variety of social theories put forth to describe or cast blame for these trends, my sense is that the increased mechanization themes of society are not helping matters. It is as if this technical and robotic reality of today, if not to blame, at least creates a reinforced environment where our social values continue to spiral out of control. People *are* more vulnerable today, and at greatest risk are those who are at the margins of society — people who are different. Quite simply, if similarity is valued, difference or diversity will be devalued.

Although this mechanization affects us all, time and time again, people who are different are caught in a more challenging web. Because of their difference, they are ferreted out, assigned to an effort to promote and produce uniformity, and kept at bay until they are ready to fit in. In a sense, the march toward uniformity and antisepticity abhors difference. It rejects and scorns difference. This mechanization sees no value for people who are different and if they can't fit in the result is rejection, isolation, stigma, or intolerance.

Yet, in a very real sense, we are all different. Sometimes we can mask, adjust, or edit our differences to fit in to the uniformity. Other times, we cannot. In the times we cannot, any of us can run the risk of a variety of actions. Most are devaluing or penalizing.

This book is, in part, an examination of difference. It is a personal and somewhat cultural exploration of difference: What it means? How it is defined? What revolves from it? By looking around, through my lens in human services, as a student, a teacher, a parent, and community member, I have assembled a review of difference. However, know as you look at this, that it does not pretend to be a firm academic or definitive work, although it is rooted from many known and respected theories. It is simply one man's assemblage of a phenomena difference, that has relevance to us all.

If the notion of difference does not fit with our technical realities and that different people are at greater risk today, then we have only three simple choices. One is to do nothing and allow things to continue as they are. The second option is to try to fix or change the difference to fit into our current realities. The third option is to look inward and push ourselves to get beyond difference.

As I think about these options, I feel we must reject the first one. To do nothing is to give up. The second notion, that of changing the different person, must also be limited. Although some people can be fixed, the majority of different people in our society will remain different. To try to fix or change these people is not only frustrating, but intolerant of difference.

I feel that the only real option for us today is to understand difference, look inward at the core of our values, and then to practice what I feel are the five step stones that can get us beyond difference.

The first section this book attempts to define difference and examine its inward and outward vestiges. In a conversational style, the effects of difference are also explored, and more specifically, how our society and its institutions have dealt with difference. It is important to note that the mechanization mentioned earlier in this preface, in a generic way, applies to the human service system as well, and often in very specific ways. The section then concludes with a crisp examination of the societal impact of difference, a pecking order that emerges, and the extent to which people can be distantiated.

However, to only explore a topic such as difference, is not enough. If we live in a world that is marching to the tune of uniformity, yet we know that we are a growing multi-cultural society, then to examine the differences that divide us is not enough. We must do more. That is why I've titled this work, *Beyond Difference*. This book goes further.

The second section of this work attempts to do just that — to get beyond difference by taking an inward turn. That is, if our march to uniformity has been driven, in part, by our rational, logical, accountable drive for precision and predictability, then it seems that the springboard beyond difference is found in the other part of our essence — our spirit and our *souls*. When I use the word soul, know that I am not making a theological statement. Rather, I see the concept of "soul" as the point of our common spirituality. In fact, I endorse the definition of "soul" developed by Thomas Moore in his book, *Care of the Soul* (1992). He states:

> Soul is not a thing, but a quality or dimension of experiencing life and ourselves. It has to do with depth, value, relatedness, heart and personal substance. (p. 5)

All the great thinkers and philosophers agreed that we are a composite of body and soul. Jefferson, in one of his famous writings, talked about the debate between his head and his heart. Einstein concluded that all measures are blunt if not balanced by the spirit. Homer's *Odyssey* examines the notion of the soul and fatherhood. Over and over, in powerful classic works, as well as simple folksy stories, the notion of spirit and soul are written into the fabric of humanity. We *are* composites of body, mind, and soul. We have this unique and difficult to define element of spirit embedded in us. To think that we don't or attempt to mechanize us as a computer (our brain) and machine (our body) is not only absurd, but terribly limiting. We are so much more as human beings and we must factor this element of spirit back into the equation.

And so the second section of *Beyond Difference* speaks more to a notion of "secular spiritualism." This is the part of our spirit that are relevant to the common good. It is not a theological, but a shared sense of the spirit, one that links us in bond with our fellow citizens and united us as humans.

In the years that I have been focusing my thoughts on secular spiritualism, I have arrived at five traits I feel are critical to getting beyond difference. Certainly, as you look these traits over, you will think of others and wonder why they haven't been included. For that question, I don't have a good answer — only that these five themes all struck a cord with me and stood the test of both formal and informal inquiry. They are related yet unique, simple yet complex. The five traits I have identified are kindness, hospitality, generosity, compassion, and forgiveness. In many regards, these five notions are connected and build upon each other, yet when examined more deeply they equally can stand alone. Each one is reviewed from a number of angles.

Also know that I have not assembled these traits and explored them in a scientific way. Yes, I did explore some scholarly works, but felt more driven to hear out everyday people on these matters. And so, I asked around and raised questions in the most unlikely places — with people I know and some I hardly know. At conferences, during coffee breaks, on airplanes, at dinner parties, with all different type of people who have had diverse experiences.

And what fun I had. Can you imagine the reaction to a question on generosity while sitting in an airport bar with people I did not know. Yet, some of these discussions were the most illuminating. One fellow even bought me a drink, although I think he felt more guilt about my question than being truly generous.

Another interesting experience was at a restaurant in Clearwater, Florida. As some friends and I batted around the notion of kindness, an older gentleman sitting near us, could not resist the urge to chime in. Before long, he was driving the discussion and his insights were fascinating.

For a full week, while at the beautiful waters of Whale Head Beach, North Carolina, my family and I shared a beach home with three other families. Every night, our dinners were peppered with great discussions. That challenging notion of forgiveness, however, etched the most lines for me.

Another discussion, at a gaming table in Las Vegas of all places, created a surrealistic scene as six gamblers musing on the concept of compassion between hands. I still remember the dealer saying to me, "will you kindly make your play, sir." I guess reflective discussions on compassion don't happen often at a blackjack table.

Family members, on both mine and my wife's side, offered many thoughts, but Aunt Dolly helped most with hospitality. It's uncanny what can be learned over a spaghetti dinner when minds and spirits ignite.

All over, people were warm and open. It almost felt like my questions opened up a ground swell for most people. They were quick to offer thoughts and seemed to delight in the more spiritual examination of life. Some peoples' responses were simple and concrete — others were incredibly deep and abstract. Many guided me to books, articles, tapes and videos they felt to be illuminating; and I followed most of these leads. A good portion of the bibliography section of this book reflects these resources. It's amazing what you can learn when you really allow your heart and spirit to listen.

This book is designed so that you need not read it from front to back. As it examines difference, I invite you to read it differently. You might be inspired to look at the section on generosity, perhaps to get some tips on getting free drinks in bars. Go ahead now, to that section. I do hope, though, that you have opportunity to look through the whole of the book. It is written in a softer style, one that readers of my first book, *Interdependence*, told me was engaging. I hope you'll feel the same with this work.

I have also assembled and inserted a number of quotes. People who know of my work, or have heard my talks, know that I am a lover of quotes. They megaphone an entire concept in a handful of words. I hope you enjoy them.

Although this book was stimulated by the many questions posed to me by people wanting to know more about interdependence, it is not designed as a "how to" or a "self help" book. I am convinced that to practice and live a life consistent with interdependence is to first look inward. However, *Beyond Difference* does pose regular and steady questions of us. It tries to push us forward by taking an inner route.

In some ways, *Beyond Difference* is the segue in a trilogy. *Interdependence* set the framework. *Beyond Difference* attempts to liberate us inside and my next book, *Strategies for Change* (still on the drawing board) pushes outward. But I'm getting ahead of myself.

So thanks for taking the time and interest in looking at this work. I was liberated in writing it and I hope you are inspired in reading it.

Al Condeluci
McKees Rocks, PA

Acknowledgments

Acknowledgments

To a large extent, I am a soloist. Although I enjoy groups and am a highly social person, I derive great satisfaction when I do something well, on my own. I seem to write better, am more creative, when I sit alone. I enjoy playing sports or games that allow me to derive my own conclusions. I'm a runner, skier, tennis, and racquetball player, all soloist sports.

Indeed, writing, to a large degree, is a soloist activity. After all the discussions and research, it boils down to one person, one pen and a weaving of ideas. This is soloist stuff.

Yet all the greatest of soloists would be naught, if it weren't for other people. And so too, *Beyond Difference* could not have happened without a myriad of others, all helpful in the weaving of this solo.

In my book, *Interdependence*, I set out to try, as frail as it was, to acknowledge people who were instrumental in helping me with that work. As I developed my list, it turned into five full pages of names. My friends, in fact, teased me about this, especially those that I failed to name. One friend thought that I must have made up some of those names as I surely could not have that many friends. As I look at it now, I guess it was a bit much.

Still, how does one do a true acknowledgment to the many people who made *Beyond Difference* happen. To shorten the list, at the risk of a new wave of teasing, I have pared down my acknowledgments to three groups: my family, my work family, and my editors.

First, to GR Press/St. Lucie Press, Dennis McClellan, and Stephanie Murphy. Thanks for your flexibility, openness, and support. I know that my work represents to a large degree, a departure from the flow and style of your publishing house. Thanks for taking the risk.

Next, my work family. For 22 years now, I have been associated with UCP of Pittsburgh. It is a dynamic, creative organization that I love with all my heart. Indeed, when I tell people I've been at UCP for 22 years they are dumbfounded that anyone can stay at one place so long. It's a shame they don't know UCP.

A deep debt of gratitude goes to my management colleagues: Tom Cloherty, Mary Lou Busby, Mary Buckholtz, Jan Bayfield, Dan Rossi, and Darla Lynn. As UCP and these folks create the bed of interdependence, so too have they carried the ball as I have been called to travel here and there. They are creative thinkers, managers, and friends, all.

So too, in my UCP family, I must thank Irene Nelson and the whole of the UCP Board of Directors. I would like to list all 30 of you but suffice it to say that your steady support has been the spark to allow the fire in me to burn.

The last note of UCP... Thanks fall with those who have offered me technical support with this project. To Carol Litzinger and Edie Scales who prepared the mainstay of the manuscript, and Beth O'Kain, who prepared the finishing touches, and Dan Rossi, who sheperded the effort. Thanks for your regular availability and thoughtful support.

And finally, to my closest, Liz, Dante, Gianna, and Santino, the band of merry souls and the keepers of my inspiration. The love and intensity I feel for you pushes my ability to describe. Liz is the rock, she keeps us all steady and together. Dante is our springboard, he keeps the key constantly turned. Gianna is the spark, with that contagious smile, always keeping us up. And Santino — ah Santino, he's the light. His innocence keeping us all on course.

And to many others, thank you all for the ideas, focus, and energy. *Beyond Difference* couldn't have happened without you!

Introduction
Interdependence and Culture

I believe in the essential unity of all people and for that matter, of all that lives. Therefore, I believe that if one person gains spiritually, the whole world gains, and if one person falls, the whole world falls to that extent.

Gandhi

Introduction
Interdependence and Culture

In 1991, I published the book, *Interdependence: The Route to Community* (2nd edition in 1995). This book was a culmination of 20 years of thinking, searching, debating, meeting, planning, and attempting to execute actions and services for people with differences brought on by disabilities. In many ways, *Interdependence* was a cathartic effort to understand, explain, introduce, define, and inspire us to a new generation of services for people who fall into the margins of society.

The major premise of *Interdependence* suggests that the formal approaches our society has taken to address the social ills brought on by difference are not working. They (our services) and organized actions are often predicated on the medical/expert model that the person with difference is not whole and must be fixed through some social/medical effort in order to be reestablished in communities or enhance their personal life.

Interdependence explores the roots of this medical/expert influence and offers example after example of the ways this model is limiting, and, at times, damaging to the very persons it is designed to serve. Four major themes are identified that remain seminal to medical/expert paradigm and are found in most organized human service systems today. These are:

- Focus on deficits
- Congregative and segregative services
- Controlled by experts
- Attempt to fix or change the focus person

These four themes are so deeply rooted into the fabric of our human service system that they are often beyond question. When I have opportunity to meet with groups to discuss these trends, many people cannot see how these four themes can be damaging. The tradition and infiltration of these concepts as core to human services work is deeply etched into the mental models that people hold.

Further, and perhaps even more penetrating, is the fact that most people in our communities today are also caught up in the same notions. That is, as our formal systems have grown up around these four themes, community has come to see them as the way it is, and the way it should be. People in our communities have bought the approach that people with difference are better off with each other under the "care" of experts. So the conditioning effect is broad and powerful.

The concept of *Interdependence* challenges these four themes. It attempts to show that when systems build around the medical/expert model, not only are there limitations, but the wedge between people with difference and the community at large, widens. In a simple sort of way, this is not hard to see. If the methodology to address, lets say mental retardation, is to identify these people's deficits, then to

We cannot leave the trap until we know we are in it.
M. Ferguson

send them to a specialty program to help them learn how to get along, have it all managed by people with degrees who know about mental retardation, then try to change them to fit in. Is it any wonder why the community might be confused when we talk about formal and informal inclusion opportunities? How are we consistent as a human service system when the way we try to include is to exclude and train?

The bold reality is that many people who have a difference, no matter what its emanation or manifestation, are probably going to remain different, despite all of the training or efforts to fix or change. This is not to suggest that people can not grow, change, or get better at some things. Of course we can and do. Rather, I am suggesting that, in some cases, maybe even most cases, people will be who they are —and is this so bad?

In some regard, there is an arrogance to our current human service system that needs to be identified and exposed. This is the system's propensity to want people to fit in, to be like us, whatever that might be. Often, we find the system telling people what their problem is, why this is bad, and then what they need to do to eradicate the problem and be like us.

This is why *Interdependence*, focuses on four different themes that promote a sense of similarity rather than difference. They are:

- Focus on capacity
- Promote relationship through inclusion
- Action revolves around focal person
- Promotes micro and MACRO change

Now when I wear my sociologist cap, I know that all people want to belong, and a major way to belonging is through being similar. The more we might manifest appearance, actions, and behaviors that are similar, the less we threaten each other, then the more we might be accepted. Although the human service system tries to change different people to be alike, another route to similarity is through people's capacities. Indeed, when people gather around a similar interest or need, differences can drift away.

When we stop to really think about it, we are, despite our many differences, incredibly similar. All of us, people of different cultures, ages, abilities and situations, share so much more than the ways we differ. In fact, in their intriguing book, *Shadows of a Forgotten Ancestor*, (1992), Carl Sagan and Ann Druyan build the case of our similarity and interdependence. They state:

We humans hold at least 99.9% of our DNA sequences in common. We are far more closely related to one another than we are to any other animal. By the similarity standards, we use in other matters, humans – even of the most disparate cultures and ethnic origins – are essentially identical in our heredities. Of the immense number of possible beings, realized and unrealized, we all are cut from the same cloth, made on the same pattern, granted the same strengths and weaknesses, and will ultimately share the same fate. Given the reality of our mutual interdependence, our intelligence, and what is at stake, are we really unable to break out of behavior patterns evolved to benefit our ancestors of long ago? (p. 415)

Now this is pause to consider. If we indeed are all similar and much more alike than different, then why all the attention to difference? Why are we trying to force people to look, act and be according to some standard norm? Why all the focus on deficits and problems, especially for those whose difference is permanent? Is it possible that this action might work against people's inclusion into the fabric of society? These are questions we must address.

Another point alluded to in *Interdependence* and clearly a key factor in understanding difference is the notion of mechanization of organizations. It is my contention that the march toward specialization, predictability, and uniformity have cut a clear theme of organizational mechanization. Most of the human service organizations I know are being pulled toward a uniformity of structure and function. Driven by wage and hour laws, union pressures, EEOC issues, accreditation standards and the like the pressure is on to conform. It's as if one type of standard should drive us all.

This type of mechanization not only creates a corporate culture that one type of approach is best and devalues groups who do not subscribe, but also leaves deep marks on all of us as individuals. This individual scarring may be the most damaging effect of mechanization.

As the book *Interdependence* attempted to address these questions, a logical theme emerged. If there are some things about people who are different that can not (or should not) be changed, then what CAN be done to facilitate their inclusion into the fabric of community so they can belong? It's a good question with a couple simple perspectives – either we change others to become more accepting of the person's difference, or focus attention on the points of our similarity.

The notion of similarity then becomes a catalyst to foster relationships with other people. Indeed, relationships become the key element to interdependence and a tangible outgrowth in our ability to get beyond difference. It's interesting to note, too, that relationships have emerged as the primary ingredient in the new scientific notion of quantum physics. Scientists who have developed quantum theories contend that relationships between entities is the key to understanding our universe. It is not the entities themselves, but how they relate and interact with each other.

The shift to quantum theory in the physical sciences was described by K.C. Cole (Wheatley, 1992) as follows:

> Most of the other giant steps in our understanding of nature were really evolutionary in that they sprang from previously established foundations, facts were reorganized, or connected in new ways, or seen in a different context. Quantum theory, however, broke away completely from those foundations, it dove right off the end. It could not (cannot) adequately be described in metaphors borrowed from our previous view of reality because many of those metaphors no longer apply. But, the net result has not been to obscure reality or make the nature of things more elusive and murky. On the contrary, most physicists would agree that what quantum theory has brought to science is exactly the opposite – concreteness and clarity. (p. 106)

More recently, the notion of quantum theory has been juxtaposed with spirituality. In a Newsweek article titled, "Science of the Scared" (Begley, 1994), references are made to the Center for Theology and the Natural Sciences in Berkeley, California. Here, new theories that link humans within the context of the universe are pondered by psychicists and theologians. Begely states:

> Even quantum mechanics, the study of subatomic interactions, offers evidence that human life and the cosmos are an interconnected whole. The eminent physicist, John Wheeler of Princeton University, refers to an observer-created universe. He means that the world does not come into being until a mind interacts with it – call it existential physics. Bizarre though it seems, for instance, measuring the spin of one subatomic particle forces a twin particle, miles away, to have the opposite spin. The observer literally creates reality, much as Eastern and other holistic faiths teach. How fitting–Lay people have to take this as a matter of faith. (pp. 56-59)

Now it seems strange to offer up an overview of quantum physics in a book that explores difference. Yet, when you stop to think about the notions of mechanization and how the intangibles of spirit and soul have been offset in our organizations, an analysis of how quantum physics is reworking natural laws of the universe can have particular relevance. Clearly, the notion of relationships is a critical variable in both organizational realities and in the laws of the universe. Taking the blending of both themes, Margaret Wheatley (1992) states:

> In the quantum world, relationships are not just interesting; to many physicists, they are all there is to reality.... In organizations, we are at the edge of this new world of relationships.... As we become more familiar with the quantum

world, a few of its organizational shapes emerge from the fog, their outlines just observable...none of us exists independent of our relationships with others. Different settings and people evoke some qualities from us and leave others dormant. In each of these relationships we are different, new in some way. (pp. 33, 34)

To this extent, the key is understanding difference is not found in the unique characteristics of the difference. To do this would be to employ an old Newtonian approach. Rather, we must focus on the ethereal qualities of the situation. We need to consider the issues of culture, values, ethics, and vision to get beyond difference.

And so, *Interdependence* concluded with some clear ideas about macroscopic change and these ethereal qualities. It examined the notions of bridge-building relationships and ways to understand community. The more informal notions about community were identified and explored. In its conclusion, *Interdependence* suggested that human services needs to spend as much time on culturing community as it does on looking at individual functioning.

> *A large part of our attitude toward things is conditioned by opinions and emotions which we unconsciously absorb as children from our environment.*
>
> A. Einstein

CULTURATION

Often, when I talk about the need to impact community and use the term "culturing," people think I mean education. As I am using it here, I see a big difference between the actions of education and culturation. To me, education is a deliberate attempt to promote a particular thesis to a particular group of people. The educator has a plan and often compliments their approach with books, materials, pamphlets, and the like. The goal is to get the audience to appreciate and then act on the new information.

Culturation, on the other hand, is a much more informal, and to a certain extent, a broader insidious process. It is about presence, and patterns and observable cues that are couched in the environment and language of the members of the culture. It is about informal leadership patterns, valued roles, and influential cultural features that lead way to an appreciation and understanding.

Often, education is antiseptic, and downward. That is, the teacher packages the information, introduces it to the student, and then tests the student retention. In fact, in more classic situations, then gauges the student to see if they "learned" the new material. With culturation, however, the process is different. It is not clear who the influencer is, and exactly when the influence might play out. As something new, such as a person or idea, is introduced to the culture, it is done so in softer ways. People just come to know through presence and constancy.

Anthropologist's call this type of learning "cultural diffusion." It relates to the process of new information or experiences becoming absorbed by the culture. Once a critical mass of people start to act on the new information, cultural learning has occurred. It is my contention that we need to think more about the process of cultural diffusion in our work than difference-related education. We must understand how new information, no matter how diverse, becomes a part of the cultural norm.

If we are to seriously harness the process of culturation as a means to inclusion of people with difference, we must understand some of its features. Over the years, anthropologists and ethologists have studied ways that clusters of species have incorporated new information or action into their patterns. One particular observation happened in Japan with macaques monkeys in the late 50s. As the story goes, a band of macaques were being observed by Japanese primatologists on an uninhabited island off the coast of Japan. As they had no natural predators (they were put there for study), the macaques became overpopulated and needed to be fed by the scientists. Weekly, sweet potatoes and wheat were airlifted in and dropped on the beach. The monkeys ate the provisions, but sand on the foodstuff surely posed a problem. Then one day, a brilliant young female, named Imo, discovered that if the sweet potatoes were dipped into a fresh water stream, the sand would disappear. In a relative period of time, the new behavior spread through the culture.

In review of this example, and influenced by many other reviews of culture diffusion, Sagan and Druyan (1992) made the following observation:

> Imo was a primate genius, an Archimedes or an Edison among the macaques. Her invention spread slowly; macaque society, like traditional human societies, is very conservative. Perhaps the fact that she (Imo) came from a high ranking family in a species given to hereditary matriarchy aided acceptance. As is usually true, adult males were the slowest to catch on, obstinate to the last; a female invented the process, other females copied her, and then it was taken up by youngsters of both sexes. Eventually, infants learned it at their mother's knee. The reluctance of the adult males must tell us something...They would rather eat sand. (p. 351)

This story, and others like it, teach us some important lessons about culturation. The point of Imo's age and social rank suggests that change is innovated, to a certain degree, by people who are sanctioned, and less vested in the status quo. It also appears that females are more open to change than males.

To a certain extent, culturation is a process that anchors because it stands the test of time. Education, on the other hand, can be manipulated or perverted in a way that it may not make a real impact on the audience. Think about this example: If I wanted a community to be more inclusive of people with disabilities is it better for me to call a town meeting and "teach" the neighbors about disability; or do I find some valued neighbors and introduce them to a person with a disability and hope the connection and presence of the person with a disability will make an impact?

Both approaches have some merit, but they also have drawbacks. Without question, education is simpler, convenient, and more easily controlled by the professional. On the down side, however, people on the receiving end of education can sometimes draw the wrong conclusions. The basic question I think we must ask is – how do communities best learn new information? This question is important because it pushes us to examine some key things about communities; things like cultural diffusion, communication patterns, and learning theories. These are the topics that are critical, not ones that focus on the difference.

Now the notions of culture, communication, and learning are ones that most people who work on behalf of those that are different fail to fully examine. Yet these three topics, and other macroscopic issues as well, are ones that I believe must be considered and understood. Those of us working toward the inclusion of those who are different must understand how cultures work, the way people communicate, and how learning occurs. Often, these three elements play out very differently in community than they do in college or some other artificial environment.

In fact, I don't think it is far off to say that most people, who work in some formal way to help people who are different move back into the mainstream, probably have some degree or certification. Indeed, the medical/expert paradigm often mandates that this be the case. This means that the lion's share of people in helping relationships are college educated or trained. I don't know about you, but my formal education was just that – formal. The curriculum was structured, I was taught by highly educated teachers, the courses revolved around jargon, the context was antiseptic and the whole experience, to a large extent, was abstract. I remember coming home from college and exposing new theories to my family and my older sister, Cathy, saying "Come on Al, get real, use words we can understand."

It has taken some time, but I finally understand what Cathy meant. She knew, to a large extent, I was out of touch with mainstream community, and it is my contention that most of us who formally attempt to help, indeed can be out of touch. We use abstract and often intellectual approaches in trying to help people understand difference and these methods, seemingly, are just not working.

I recently did an informal survey, totally unscientific, and without any solid controls, yet still found some intriguing results. You might want to try it with your own system. At a couple of conferences where I was speaking, I asked my audiences to do a quick mental poll of their staff and come up with a percentage of those who are college educated. Keep in mind, that most of the folks in my audiences work in some form of rehabilitation in an effort to help people with disabilities get back to their communities. It is clearly a medical/expert paradigm.

In the many forums where I have done this, I have found that four out of five staff (some 80%) are college educated. Indeed, many forums had 100% who were college educated. Now, think about this – almost 100% of the staff responsible for connecting the person back to the community, are undergraduate or graduate school educated. Yet, in most communities only one out of five members (20%) are college educated. Shouldn't this discrepancy give us pause to reflect.

Now, I bring this up not to downgrade a college education, or to put down our communities for being less formally educated. I merely say this to push thinking about the way most of us in the field have been taught and in turn, how we might see the world, compared to the very world we are trying to influence. People on the street, members of the communities we hope to influence, often process information, communicate and learn differently than the typical college approach. As my sister, Cathy, said, we need to "get real."

I remember an experience a few years back when I was meeting with a tenant council on behalf of some folks with disabilities who were planning to move into the apartment complex. Using the professional, educational approach, I talked with the tenant council about disability, some of the manifestations, trying to give them good information. Before I knew it, however, some residents picked up on some minor points about head injury and blew them way out of proportion. I learned a real lesson about education and culturation that night.

Now, all of this is not to say that culturation or the ways of the street is a panacea, the total answer to the community inclusion issue. It does have its own drawbacks. One of them is the slowness and tediousness of enculturation to take hold. It is a constant presence that is necessary and this just takes time. Another challenge is the uncontrolled variables we face. Culturation mandates that the community be in charge, not we as professionals. Many of us have problems being out of the driver's seat.

Still, despite these drawbacks, in my mind culturation offers the best alternative to the inclusion challenge. We must look seriously at this approach, study and understand community, and then give it our best. People of communities are the real gatekeepers to opening the doors to others, not the professionals. We must learn how to culture community.

In a way, our challenge is to find ways across the "borders" we create between each other. We are indeed a multicultural society, and each of our cultures offer both elements that can lure us together or drive us apart. In his thoughtful book, culture of complaint, Robert Hughes (1993) speaks to this point:

> Multiculturalism asserts that people with different roots can coexist, that they can learn to read the image-banks of others, that they can and should look across the frontiers of race, language, gender, and age without prejudice or illusion, and learn to think against the background of a hybridized society. It proposes, modestly enough, that some of the most interesting things in history and culture happen at the interface between cultures. It wants to study bor-

der situations, not only because they are fascinating in themselves, but because understanding them may bring with it a little hope for the world...separatism rejects exchange. (pp. 87-88)

A final note on culturation, is that culture offers a composite picture. Each of us, in some type of critical mass, creates a flow of the culture. So when we talk about culturing community, I am really suggesting that we examine our individual beliefs and actions. Our culture is a mirror of us, and if we don't like the current flow of culture, then we must start with each of us. To some extent, this simple notion is both exciting and challenging. That is, if a cultural reaction to difference concerns us, then we must first augment our own behavior in the matter. Chances are that we may be guilty of the very problems of which we complain.

> *Interdependence is a wider paradigm, and with a wider paradigm there are no enemies. We are not liberated until we liberate others.*
>
> *M. Ferguson*

TOWARD INTERDEPENDENCE

In the brief time since the publication of *Interdependence*, I have been amazed by its impact and receptivity. As I write these words, the book has now gone to a second edition with a strong showing in both United States and Canada and recent introduction in England and Europe. It is being used at a number of universities and colleges and has been incorporated in hundreds of conferences. People who have read or heard the concept presented, call or write me almost daily to talk more. I have conducted more in-service training and program audits than I can count, and as of the publication of this book some 15,000 people have been exposed to this concept. Clearly, *Interdependence* is making a mark.

All of this has been rewarding and flattering, but the basic question remains; how can we make interdependence happen in our agencies, organizations, schools or our personal lives? People I meet with, especially when they have time to really engage the theory, want to know how to do it. How can we really get beyond difference?

As I have been pressed with these questions, I have been tempted to come up with some quick prescription, the formal answer to the question. In fact, isn't this just what the medical/expert paradigm expects; that the specialist comes up with the answer?

Indeed, I must confess, early on, I did try to give people the answer. Using a thrust bore more from a Newtonian perspective, I told them to examine their organization's mission and vision statement, to look at their agency literature, to make sure that the symbols of their work were validating and consistent with the principles of *Interdependence*. I have suggested that those dealing with difference focus on capacities rather than deficits, to find people's tickets to commonality. All of these, and other ideas I have advanced, have been honest attempts to get people to not only think, but to act, as well.

At this point, however, I am beginning to reassess my posture on the question of how to do interdependence. I am becoming increasingly sensitive to the fact that one can not really do interdependence, just the same as one can not really do any other type of philosophical notion. This is not to say that actual behaviors that are consistent with interdependence can not occur. Of course they can and should. I am beginning to feel, however, that they are not some prescriptive behaviors, but actions more of the heart than of the mind.

My posture today about interdependence swirls more from the notion of spirit than of intellect. In fact, in many of my presentations I use the framework of spiritual secularism as a base line for "doing" interdependence. In these talks, I advance themes of spirit rather than clinical points of intervention. This perspective is captured more in the quantum notions that lack uniformity and are hard to predict or control.

When I speak of the spiritual dimension, again, know that I am not using the term in a theological way. By spiritual, I mean the way we all experience life, the intangibles of being appreciated, accepted, and acknowledged. All of us have spiritual dimensions that we share and these often are the things that bond us as humans. In 1990, the Task Force on Self-esteem, established in California to

> *We have a spiritual longing for community and relatedness and for a cosmic vision, but we go after them with literal hardward instead of with sensitivity of the heart.*
> *Thomas Moore, 1992*

examine the social problems of drugs, gangs, and violence concluded that one reason for these ills was a loss of spirit. They defined spirituality as experiencing ourselves in relationship to the universe. This definition captures my understanding of spirit and how I use it in this work.

It is interesting to note that even when spirituality is encased in the world of religion a sense of devaluation has occurred. Steven Carter (1993) articulated this notion in *The Culture of Disbelief* when he stated:

> More and more, our culture seems to take the position that believing in the tenets of one's faith represents a kind of mystical irrationality, something that thoughtful, public-spirited American citizens would do better to avoid .... We are trying, here in America, to strike an awkward but necessary balance, one that seems more and more difficult with each passing year... One result is that we often ask our citizens to split their public and private selves, telling them in effect that it is fine to be religious in private, but there is something askew when those private beliefs become the basis for public action. (pp. 6-8)

Although Carter doesn't argue for more church spirituality, he does point out clearly how America has embraced a culture of disbelief and how the "public square" now has no room for spiritual discussions.

Over the past few months, as I have thought more about the interdependence question and spirituality, I am struck by the cultural issues. Most of us appreciate the theological aspects of spirituality, but to truly push spiritual issues into the secular world requires that we think about culture.

A Newsweek cover story titled, *In Search of the Sacred* (Nov. 28, 1994) explored how spiritual elements have become reinvigorated within the culture. They (Kantrowitz et al.) state:

> Americans have always been a religious people, of course. Even during the past several decades, when it seemed like the prevailing culture was overwhelmingly irreverent and secular, legions of the faithful filled pews every Sunday. But for the baby boomers in particular, spirituality was off the radar scope. Instead, as a generation, boomers embraced political activism, careerism, even marathon running, with an almost religious zeal. Now, it's suddenly OK, even chic, to use the 'S' words – soul, sacred, spiritual, and sin. In a Newsweek, poll, a majority of Americans (58%) say they feel the need to experience spiritual growth. And a third of all adults report having had a mystical or religious experience. (pp. 53-54)

If we pause to look more deeply at this aspect of spirituality within the culture there is an interesting history. Probably, the first person to examine American culture and identify this notion of collective spirit was Alexis de Tocqueville in his penetrating book, *Democracy in America* (1848). As a student of societies, de Tocqueville spent a few years travelling and analyzing America. He was looking for nuances that set our society apart from Europe. One of his observations was the propensity in America for the development of community associations designed to solve problems or meet goals. These associations were informally structured and driven by common goodwill. This more spiritual sense of organizing for the common good, to a certain extent, was born from our rural roots and pioneer notions. They fused together to create what de Tocqueville called "habits of the heart." These "habits" were both practical and spiritual.

In an interesting sociological follow-up, Robert Bellah (1985) examine how America has changed since Tocqueville's visit and writing. Their review and speculation on changes was reported in their book, aptly titled, *Habits of the Heart.* Among other reasons, Bellah et al. suggest that our spiritual notions have slowly eroded since the mid 1800s. They report that the mechanization and isolation, created during the industrial revolution, led to a tired and vulnerable population. Although most of those influenced by these industrial changes were people who lived in urban areas, these people began to shift the collective perspective. Rather than be responsible to each other, workers turned inward and expected government and services to watch out for society.

> *Diversity is a source of strength and balance. We add to our lives when we appreciate and accept the cultural and ethnic differences in our society.*
> *CFTR, 1990*

In the years that followed, other influences occurred, but the march toward specialization and homogeneity was well on its way. To a certain extent, as industrialization brought isolation in the work place, it also brought more money to the worker. With more money in hand, there was more ability to buy what one needed, rather than to rely on associations. These trends led to people looking inward, rather than outward toward others.

As I think about de Tocqueville's work and Bellah's analysis, I am drawn to explore this notion of homogeneity and heterogeneity. Although we consider ourselves as a heterogeneic society, most of our patterns are homogeneic. We tend to spend time with and relate to people who are often very much like us. Although it can fuel a sense of security, this propensity, I believe affects more our habits of the heart, and in turn, our spirituality. That is, if unchecked, it causes us to push away from people who are different from us.

We become less interested in others and begin to reject or even fear diversity.

It seems to me, however, that the major elements of our spirituality are about just the opposite – understanding and respecting diversity. If most of our societal patterns are to remain homogeneic, thus resulting in less opportunity to see difference, this can lead to suspicion, and retreat from those we perceive as different. This fear and retreat then, can clearly dampen or stunt our spirituality and openness.

Another point in this review of spirituality, revolve around dependence and independence. We all have this drive to be independent, to control our environment and be autonomous. Yet, the ultimate aspect of independence is to be totally autonomous. In its strongest sense this means virtual isolation. We have this picture of the strong independent person who can do it all themselves, yet a totally independent person needs no one else.

In fact, it seems that the dominance of independence has caused our society to have a phobia about dependence. People's fear of dependence is legion. Parents are telling their adult children that they do not want to be a burden on them, as if an adult child taking care of an aging parent is abnormal. Further, more and more younger adults are creating "living wills" to dictate that they do not want to live in a state of dependence. Indeed, as I write these words, Dr. Jack Kovorkian, the dubbed "suicide doctor," has participated in yet another assisted death. His patient indicated she did not want to be a burden on her family.

Surely today, though, we know two key things in this debate around independence. One is that none of us are totally capable of independence. All of us, to a greater or lesser degree, need other people. We have dependencies that can only be solved through other people. The other point is that through relationships and diversity we find richness in our own lives. We know that a blending of diverse people create a powerful synergy. In fact, if we are successful in our lives it is because of other people around us. The key is not independence, but interdependence.

So how do we make interdependence happen? I believe that it can not happen until we examine our own spirituality. We must take the time to look deeper into who we are, what we believe and how we can open our own hearts. We have to honestly appraise how the medical/expert model might have conditioned us to be calculating and clinical, and how the march to mechanization have, to a certain extent, stripped our souls.

In his book, *The Presentation of Self in Everyday Life* (1959), Erving Goffman wrote about our public and private lives. He described how people in society tend to draw a line between the public actions and private affairs. This dichotomy has created a split between the professional, more calculated self and the private, more spiritual side.

Most of us can relate to this public/private face reality. It seems as if we're all held accountable to act one way publicly and quite another privately. This is not necessarily bad unless the values between the two worlds differ. That is, if in your private side you show spiritual actions to family and friends, but in your public side you are calculating and aloof, there will not only be discourse in behavior, but basic humanity needs of the public side will suffer. Although Goffman's perspective on the public/private issue is more than 30 years old, it seems that the rift in these two worlds is greater today than ever before. People, especially those in highly visible positions, seemingly kept a close lid on their private lives so as to not have their public life affected.

Although this line of demarcation plays out in many areas, one interesting point of observation is found in the world of politics. Reporters today, dig deeply into candidates private lives for possible blemishes that can lead to a story. This has caused most politicians to closely guard their private affairs or to lead a totally public life. Again, this may not necessarily be bad unless a hostile, or calculating side dominates. A tragedy here is when a candidate shows a softer, more human side and the behavior is then perceived as weak. In the 1992 Clinton/Bush election, the incumbent, then President Bush, was advised to come out strong, to attack candidate Clinton's character, to show he (Bush), was the stronger of the two.

Now clearly, there are, and, to a certain extent should be, differences between our public and private lives. People can not always be on display or in the public eye. We all need room to relax. My concern with the dichotomy, however, is when we let our spiritual notions play out in only one side. That is, if people feel their spiritual self should only be dominant in their private lives, then we run the risk that spirituality will be lessened, or non existent in their public life. This is not only a tragedy, but creates a harsh and cruel world.

The public/private debate around spiritualism raises some serious questions, as well. To a large extent, the framework of our constitution in the United States speaks to the separation of church and state. Now, in the purest sense, this means the separation between organized theology and government. This is obviously a positive distinction as it relates to democracy because it prevents one type of religion to become legally dominant. The concern it might raise, however, is when we confuse spiritualism with theology. As I stated earlier, the notion of spiritualism is a holistic concept, one that is not tied to any type of theology, although spiritual messages are found in all organized theologies. The spiritualism that roots this work are notions that must be present in our public, as well as our private lives. When we add hospitality, generosity, kindness, compassion, or forgiveness into the equation of our public lives we are NOT imposing theology, but promoting a spiritual respect for one another.

An interesting lens to observe spiritual issues that drift into public domain is found in today's formal human services. As I pointed out in *Interdependence*, most of our organized approaches to dealing with difference today are driven by a medical/expert model. Although there are many clarifying points of the medical model, one important notion is that of scientific, antiseptic prediction. Further, the influences of Newtonian science keeps us harnessed to mechanics. Most medical models have little room for spiritual issues, and if they do it is usually an afterthought or a lesser valued aspect.

This point is driven home in many examples, and more recently has been picked up in the arts and literature. In the 1991 movie release, *The Doctor*, the Academy Award winning actor, William Hurt plays a hugely successful heart surgeon who has no use for the human/spiritual variables. In early scenes, he chastises his residents for getting too close to patients. He speaks to the clutter and emotionality that can get in the way and cloud the surgeon's objectivity. Then he comes down with throat cancer and becomes a patient himself. He finds himself treated by a medical specialist who harbors the same feelings of objectivity. Of course, an epiphany occurs and Hurt changes his entire perspective.

Another popular example of the importance of the spiritual variables in human services is found in the writings of Dr. Bernie Siegel. With his popular book, *Love, Medicine, and Miracles* (1989), Siegel tells story after story of how spiritual factors made dominant differences in the lives, and often, the recovery of his patients.

It seems to me that you can not really engage in human services, or any other type of people oriented business for that matter, without a prominent place for the spiritual dimensions. One without the other seems impossible. Yet, the specialization models of our businesses pushes us constantly toward the more predictive, scientific side of the equa-

> *The man who evaluates, oversimplifies and thereby falsifies living reality*
> *Ortega Y. Gasset*

tion. For example, when I am doing workshops on interdependence, I often get asked questions like "how can we measure inclusion for people with disabilities?" Now, it seems to me, that you really can not truly measure the notion of inclusion. How does one know if they are included in a group? Just being *in* a group is not tantamount to being of a group. Yet, people in human services tell me that they must be able to put things into units of service and must be able to measure their work or they stand to lose funding. Now to me, this propensity to focus on the need to measure and predict is yet another example of the skewing of human services toward the medical model. This is not to say that a human service program should not be accountable. They should, but we must find ways to allow and validate the spiritual, less predictable side of any type of service to have equal value.

Still, it seems that pure scientists are constantly finding ways to lessen the importance of spiritual things that can not be predicted as readily. This is why the hard, or more pure sciences, such as chemistry and physics, have been elevated to a higher sense of validity (through precision and control of variables) than the social science research that is performed. It is as if the pure sciences are more academic and predictable, therefore more respected.

Rivalry and cruelty thrive on distance because distance allows us to turn people into abstractions.

A. Kohn

The march of this type of pressure continues to push social science researchers, and to a lesser extent, human service professionals, to be more accountable and predictive in their work. The net effect of these pressures then is the devaluation of the spiritual/intangible side of services. That is, people who work in human services, or more specifically, promote the spiritual side of the business, are not thought to be as efficacious.

The approach of professionalism, and to certain degree, clinical distance from people who receive human services, is one that most students of human services learn as routine. I remember in the Graduate School of Social Work, being encouraged to carry myself as a professional. Although there may be a number of interpretations to what this means, I recall the context as suggesting that we keep objective on issues. "Don't get too close, as you might lose your professional perspective," was the nature of the message.

Now, I don't know about others, but I can not see myself truly doing my current work without being subjective, getting close to the people I know. How else might I get a sense of another's struggles and perspective if I don't become subjective. This leads to a sense of empathy, attempting to "feel" another person's reality. I believe this can not be done without getting close.

Yet, the stuff of our existing human service systems today is more that of "we/they." And most of the "we's" are light years away from the "they's." Indeed, the physical features in the facilities used to serve people who have some difference, show clear signs of who is who and which players are welcomed where. Staff have their designated places and the "clients," theirs.

This "we/they" reality affects other points, as well. If the professionals of human services keep a "we" distance from the people they serve, then their ability to truly understand, and speak with and for people, will be affected. This is especially true if the people served have difficulty speaking for themselves. If professionals remain aloof and "professional," how can they really advocate effectively? Knowing about people through books and readings is a far cry from being *with* people in their life situation.

> Not I, but the world says it:
> All is one.
>
> Heraclitus

It is interesting to me, that the typical outlet of people who are different is often some formalized human service. Note that *human* is the operative word in the phrase, "human service." The implication is that the services rendered will be humane. That is, they will be sensitive to the nuances of people in general and will endeavor to accept diversity.

Yet today, human service is riddled with terms and influences that sometimes makes me wonder if we can keep the spirit of humanity. We hear talk about "units" of services, or "slots" to be filled. Time and time again, human service professionals talk about new "technologies" to be clinically applied to their clients. Management by objectives (MBO) has become a dominant way of thinking about what services should be rendered. Increasing specialization has created highly trained technicians that are detailed in one particular field, but have little appreciation in most other areas. Further, services themselves have parceled into particular domains that only look at one need area.

These and other trends are clear signs of the drifting of humaneness and spiritual notions of today's human services. In fact, probably the most visible signal of this mechanization of human services is found when one examines conference and in-service training topics. Usually, the standard fare in my field at conferences is highly specialized and focused material that is either technical or clinical to the difference in question. That is, if the conference revolves around a topic such as traumatic head injury, the bevy of workshops are sure to be technical to brain dysfunction.

I am particularly sensitive to this phenomena as in 1994 alone, I addressed over 30 different conference gatherings in the disability field. Often, my topic (the concept of interdependence), which is a values-based discussion, is the only philosophical item on the agenda. Similarly, most agency in-service topics tend to be technical or clinical.

Now it is curious to me, that if human services are about both the spiritual as well as the technical aspects of addressing difference, why don't we have more focus on spiritual aspects? The answer to the question is found woven through most of what was previously exposed in *Interdependence*. It has to do with the march of medicalization, the prominence of the scientific model, the devaluation of spiritual information, the focus of Newtonian science, the mechanization of services and the deep rooted "we/they" notions of professionalization. We must balance the equation and look at spiritual issues.

This book does just this. It turns attention to the human side of addressing difference. Rather than examine technical, expert ways to help people, it speaks more to helping ourselves open up to others. If we are ever to truly get beyond difference as a society, we must first look inward, person to person. Things won't change until we change, and we won't change until we push ourselves spiritually.

Thus, the answer to the question, "How do we do interdependence," must be explored first from the spiritual side. If interdependence is about looking beyond difference and into our souls, we must think about the "stuff" of our spirits. How open and receptive and welcoming are we? In human services, we rarely look at this side of ourselves, yet interdependence can not happen until we do.

So, lets move on in this journey. In the spirit of openness, let's turn first to the phenomena of difference.

It is impossible to be ignorant of the end of things if we know their beginnings.

Thomas Aquinas

SECTION I

∽ DIFFERENCE ∽

1

Difference: An Overview

Here hills and valleys,
*   the woodland and the plain*
Here earth and water seem to
*   strive again*
Not chaos—like together
*   crushed and bruised*
But as the world harmoniously
*   confused*
Where order in variety we see, and
*   where, all things differ, all agree.*

Alexander Pope

1

Difference: An Overview

It can start innocently, or it can start explosively. You might not invite it, or you can be seeking it. It might come at your hands, or it could be from the hands of others. But when it comes, you will know it.

I'm talking about difference. The state of being seen, or feeling or knowing that you are different from the majority of other people in your network. Difference can come in all shapes and form. Some people are different in appearance, or skin color, or culture. Others are different in the way they think, or act, or relate. Still others are different because they are poor, inept, or unhealthy; tall, short or squat.

Difference alone is not necessarily cause for negative experiences, hostility, or rejection. There are situations where difference can lead to a valued or esteemed state. For example, in our society today, athletes, especially those who excel in their sport, may be highly valued. Their difference in skill and mastery is cause for adulation. Still, the notion of difference is usually experienced from its shadow side. When someone asserts that they feel different it is usually a statement that they feel bad, lonely, or isolated.

Difference is something that we all have known or felt. Somewhere in our lives, we have been the odd person out and in this regard, anyone reading this book has felt some vestiges of difference. Like the time you were not selected for a part you wanted in a play or a job that you knew you could do. How about the times you wanted to be with or among a group, but were not welcomed into the fold. The times no one danced with you, or the times no one called.

These experiences, when we care to dig them up, push the remembrance of difference. When you are positioned as someone who is different or odd, the feelings of distantiation and rejection can become intense. This is especially true when the experiences happen at periods in your life when you are more susceptible, such as when you are entering a new group, or moving into a new experience, or at a tender age. These situations can make one feel not only odd, but alien.

I remember a clarifying experience of being different that led to an alien perspective. In the early 70s, I was invited to a conference that was exploring disability and society's treatment of people with disabilities. The topic was one I had examined in other forums, but this one was markedly different. The conference was sponsored by the Berkeley, California Center for Independent Living, and the stark majority of the participants were people with severe disabilities. I remember seeing more types of disabilities than I had ever before. Being able-bodied, I was clearly the different party.

As people at this conference met to study oppression and disability, I couldn't help feeling that all eyes were on me. We talked about the years of oppression experienced by people with disabilities and I had that odd feeling that everyone perceived me as an oppressor. I tried hard to rationalize that these feelings were just in my head, but seemingly could not convince myself or others in the room. I was clearly different than the majority of people at this gathering and could feel the effects of difference.

This was a simple example, but one that caused me to review and then personally explore, the phenomena of difference. As I thought (and continue to think) about this concept, I found an interesting line between what I had experienced and what I had learned. As a student interested in human behavior in society, I was taught about the historic features of difference; about cultures and races and situations that made (and make) groups of people different. I remember reading classic books such as *Stigma* by Goffman (1963) and *Normalization* by Wolfensberger (1972), or more recent titles such as *Bearing the Cross* by Garrow (1986). These, and others, gave me an academic introduction to understanding difference.

On the other hand, when I found myself in a personal experience that made, or treated me as different, the softness of academic understanding was replaced with the harshness of reality. It is really amazing how the academic world of textbooks can mute the ugliness and negative feelings of oppression. I'm sure this is why groups such as the Anti-Defamation League or NAACP want people to never lose the feelings of atrocities like the holocaust, or the early stages of civil rights, the experiences of Little Rock, Arkansas, Selma, Alabama, and the other fronts of racial discrimination.

Another interesting feature between learning about something in a book or feeling it through experience is the innocence that can accompany the analysis. Books put things into a logical perspective, even if we are outraged by the situation. For example, we know that in a sick way, Hitler and his key advisors created and activated a plan to eliminate the Jews; that they perceived the Jew-

> *What we see depends on what we are prepared to see.*
> P. Senge

ish people as evil, and this was their rationalization for the holocaust. This rationalization hardly eases the depth of the pain for families who lost loved ones in this debacle, yet for others the academic perspective might seem plausible. In fact, today, some groups of people offer a revisionist version of events — as if the holocaust never really happened. When the U.S. Holocaust Museum opened in April 1993, a CBS survey found that some 24% of Americans did not believe, know or think the holocaust had ever happened.

Another similar example, is found when we look at civil rights. With the passage of time and an abstract sense of the political reality of the time seem to blend into a perspective that "boys will be boys." Yet, when you sit to watch a documentary such as the

Blackstone Production of, *Eyes on the Prize*, the horror of beatings, lynchings, and outright terrorism jump from the screen. People were victimized and brutalized and no dent of time will change that reality.

Another point for consideration, is the clear delineation between the legal perspective on difference and society's action. The best example here would be the Civil Rights Act of 1964. This antidiscriminatory legislation was legion for its time. Finally, we had a law that was to end segregation and discrimination against minorities. Yet, in the 30 years since its passage, our society is still riddled with wanton discrimination. Even though the law says discrimination is illegal we have example after example of softer more subtle forms of discrimination. Although our laws have changed, our spirit for discrimination has not.

Legal scholars and students of society are well aware of this dichotomy between the letter and spirit of the law. An astute observer of society, Alexander Solzhenitsyn stated (1973):

> A society based on the letter of the law and never reaching any higher, fails to take advantage of the full range of human possibilities. The letter of the law is too cold and formal to have a beneficial influence on society. Whenever the tissue of life is woven of legalistic relationships, this creates an atmosphere of spiritual mediocrity that paralyzes men's noblest impulses. (p. 526)

This is why any formal change of laws are not really viable until society believes the change is viable. Until this happens people will find ways to assault the letter of the law.

Indeed, it is amazing how easy it is for people to rationalize activities that are horrendous. One example that comes to mind is the "not guilty" verdict rendered in the spring of 1992 on the Rodney King case. For many people who viewed the amateur videotape of the police beating of King, the "not guilty" verdict was unbelievable. How could the 12 jury members not see the brutality of the act. Yet, over the course of the trial, as the jury saw the tape run over and over again, the horror of the clubbing turned into an antiseptic conclusion that King himself, dictated the police action. Witness after witness testified to the difference between a death blow and a restraining blow. All of this academic perspective masked the undeniable ugliness of this event.

On the feeling side, however, it is often difficult to understand or deal with the determinants of the effects of difference. For example, when I was at the disability conference, I could not understand why the participants at this gathering were rejecting me and the things I was trying to add to the conference. Even when I tried to academically understand people's behavior, it was confusing to me; a real sense of discourse. The academic perspective just didn't help.

This simple example resulted in my being shunned, and to a certain extent, rejected at this conference; but what about people who have had major brushes with difference and just cannot understand or appreciate the academic perspective? Consider:

- The person who was in a car accident and through brain damage now, has a serious cognitive challenge. In examples I have seen, persons have lost friends, lovers, employment, and dignity; all major losses. Indeed, traumatic brain injury is the major killer of people under the age of 30. For many of the close to 1.8 million people who are injured each year and survive, the difference and resulting distantiation they face is devastating. To further complicate the issue, many of the cognitive, physical, or emotional changes that result from brain injury will never be totally remedied.
- Or the family who has lost economic stability through the recession, and is now on welfare. In our day and age, this type of falling from grace can lead to lost mortgages, lost status, hunger, and possible homelessness. The resultant poverty affects health care, family stability and, almost universally, individual dignity. These are life threatening situations.

♦ Or the person that had a brush with the law, who is now trying to re-enter the job market. The degradation of being an ex-con, not only makes community reunion difficulty, but can assault one's self image and lead to the roller coaster of crime recidivism. Once a person is labeled an ex-con all the typical stereotypes follow. In our present climate of law and order, rehabilitation from a crime can be next to impossible.

♦ Or the person with retardation, who is recently deinstitutionalized from a state hospital. The isolation from life and common community experiences is not only distantiating, but stigmatic as well. People have their "picture" of people with retardation, thus the treatment that ensues is often infantile and degrading. Forget importance in the community, the options usually available and experiences that follow for people with retardation, are off setting and lowly. Yet, for most of us, the initial family and neighborhood experiences are the stepping stones to self worth, self-esteem and success.

♦ Or the person with AIDS, who knows their life will be cut short. The negative treatment and ostracism from society often makes the person's last days, their loneliest. Indeed, given the tremendous stigma attached to AIDS, this group provides a provocative example for the study of difference. Just the mere thought of someone's blood being different is enough to create a powerful distantiation. No one should have to live or die the way most people with AIDS do.

All these groups of people and those who love them, know the ravishes of being different, and the terrible stigma felt and faced by a society or community that seemingly despises, avoids or just doesn't care. The people identified in these groups are different. For most of them, their lives are changed, perhaps by their doing, maybe not. The point is, that in the wake of their difference, they are seen and treated as alien from all the rest of us. They are subjected to the biases and perceptions of society about "them." They are cast into role expectations about "their kind" and are often not given either opportunity or credit to do or be something else.

This issue of role expectation, is an important one in understanding reactions to difference. Sociologists know, and most of us have experienced situations where we have been cast into expected roles and then some predictable results occur. That is, if persons find themselves in situations that carry with them certain roles, often they will take on that role. Think of things that may have happened to you; times when people expected you to be strong at a funeral, or taking the lead at a meeting. More often than not, you probably followed the expectation.

Man is what he believes.
Anton Chekhov

Sociologists think this happens because of peer pressure and our drive to be accepted. Know, however, that role expectation has both positive and negative power, and can influence roles accordingly. We can be influenced to take on either helpful, affirmative roles, as well as destructive or hurtful behaviors if the expectations are strong enough.

Thus, when you have situations of difference, where a person has shifted from one reality to another, the expectations that surround each reality will come into play. Think for a minute of a person who is a family leader, gainfully employed, and active in community. Then one day, this person is involved in a serious accident and experiences a change to his or her current reality. The devastation of the accident leads to serious cognitive (thinking) and physical (moving) manifestations. As this person returns home, the expectations change. Given the new situation, the person might now loose his or her job, take a back seat in family decisions, and have difficulty participating in community activity.

As we analyze this example, it is important to sort out the cause of this change. Clearly, expectations set in and the individual may begin to behave the way everyone expects. This shift in behavior is a strong, and often predictable, aspect of social influence. People will react as often to expectations as they might to actual physical or cognitive complexities.

This notion of role expectation and role behavior happens in a number of ways. Often, with difference, we can see it materialize in negative ways. Daily, I come into contact with people who have had disabilities, and many of these people have given in to the script presented by the societal stereotype, that of the incapable. They have been told and reminded of their difference so long, that they have bought the script.

On the other hand, however, role behavior can have a positive effect. This will happen when the expectations are set on a higher level. A good example here is the 1980 US Olympic Hockey Team. In these games, and at this era of history, the Russians were the oppressive team to beat. The American team skated into these games with a clear difference in talent and experience, especially in comparison to the Russians. But the growing expectation that settled over Lake Placid that winter was of victory. And in the course of the two week competition, these mediocre American skaters did the impossible — they defeated the Russians. People who were there testified that the feeling of victory was everywhere, not just during the games. The role expectation was both powerful, positive, and persuasive. Everyone there, indeed, believed in miracles.

> *There is no absolute knowledge, and those who claim it, whether they are scientists or dog-matists, open the door to tragedy.*
>
> *J. Bronowski*

DIFFERENCE AND DISTANTIATION

More often than not, however, difference is devalued and people with difference fall prey to a preset of exclusion. In many cases, the person's differences can lead to a type of banishment. That is, the devaluation that is associated with being different can set up walls and barriers that are often impossible to overcome. In many situations, the different person is recommended to be with other people who have the same type of difference. This process, usually driven by experts or professionals, conditions the person and the person's family to feel it is either better, or more appropriate, to live with others of similar ilk.

In my years at UCP, I have witnessed countless examples of situations where people with disabilities and their families were convinced that keeping themselves or their family member with people of their own "kind," was (or is) the best thing to do.

Now this type of recommendation is one that cannot be quickly dismissed. It is also vital to the concept of interdependence, as the guts of this theory (interdependence) is to allow for the acceptance and connection of people with differences in community. If there is a propensity to remove people from community because they are different (and I believe there is) then an understanding of this type of action is vital to its reversal. We need to understand that although the recommendation to be with ones own kind is often made by professionals, it does represent a type of banishment. When we examine this action as a form of banishment some key features follow.

First, we must acknowledge that any type of banishment is the strongest form of punishment. More than capital punishment, past societies have used banishment as the epitome of sacrifice. Taking a life is the ultimate of suffering, but to really punish people is to have them live in loneliness and isolation to think about their crime. This is why most societies' penal systems impose solitary confinement to their most hardened criminals.

It is not a bold segue to consider some of our society's formal human services as a form of banishment. Most approaches to difference today stress a period of time to be with "your own kind." People with disabilities spend much time with other similar people as a form of "therapy." It is felt that they need to come to grips with their disabilities and peers can best help in this process. Then, when a person is ready to return to the community, a variety of self help groups are recommended. Indeed, we have developed all types of long-term groups and agencies to serve in this purpose.

From another lens, however, these actions and groups are a type of banishment, as well. As much as they help, so too can they distance the very persons that they are designed to serve. Further, as these groups have attempted to publicize their availability, they have also announced to the community that a place exists for "them," and it is a special place at that. It is no wonder that community advice for a newly disabled person is to call the Center for Independent Living, or, for the poor person, the welfare office, or, for the elderly person, the local senior citizens' center. They can help "your" kind.

If you pause for a moment and think about difference, any of the areas I mentioned earlier in this text, or many others that can be identified, there are special places for "them." Consider the following list:

Different Group	"Their" Place
Alcoholics	ONALA, AA
Retarded	ARC, Group Homes, Sheltered Work, Special Olympics
Gays	Act Up, Hospices
Poor	Welfare, Food Stamps, Subsidized Housing, Food Pantries
Seniors	AARP, Retirement Communities, Senior Centers, High Rise Homes
Disabled	CIL, Specialty Agencies (UCP, Easter Seals).

This list is not to suggest that specialty agencies designed around specific issues are not important or do not serve a valuable purpose. They are and often do. But they also have a darker side as it relates to image and the perspective of society at large. There has to be a balance to the importance and viability of specialty groups. I am concerned, however, that today they are playing more and more of an important (or even vital) place in the lives of people with difference. They are, as Burton Blatt (1981) suggested years ago, making it easy for us to banish our brothers from our midst.

As difference and distantiation spirals, the different person begins to either feel or believe that indeed they don't really belong. They start to "own" the stigma and

> I know of no more encouraging fact than the unquestionable ability of man to elevate his life by a conscious endeavor.
>
> Henry David Thoreau

inherent devaluation that follows and will often agree, or passively accept the treatment they are rendered. Many people begin to see themselves out of the lens of their difference. I've had people call me and say, "I'm a CP, can you help me?" Of course I will. After all, I work for UCP!

CONSCIOUSNESS: AN ESSENTIAL INGREDIENT

As painful as these experiences of difference can be, they can have at least one powerful, positive notion — that of enhanced consciousness. There seems to be story after story that suggest that with the pain of suffering comes an awakening of consciousness. At times, if you are a person experiencing the pains of difference, it might feel like this consciousness is not positive, especially when it leads to questions that start with "why." Like, "Why won't they give me a chance?" Or, "Why won't they accept me for who I am?" Or, "Why can't I get a date?"

This issue of consciousness, though, is an important one. In a basic way, consciousness is a mental state where people incorporate new or known information in a direct way to their actions. It is interesting that although most people have heard, or could offer a definition of consciousness, there are few formal groups or writings devoted to its study.

In his strong book, *Flow: The Psychology of Optimal Experience*, Mihaly Csikszentmihalyi (1990) takes the time to focus the concept of consciousness. He states:

> The function of consciousness is to represent information about what is happening outside and inside the organism in such a way that it can be evaluated and acted upon by the body. In this sense, it functions as a clearinghouse for sensations, perceptions, feelings, and ideas, establishing priorities among all the diverse information. Without consciousness we would still "know" what is going on, but we would have to deliberately weigh what the senses tell us, and respond accordingly. And, we can also invent information that did not exist before; it is because we have consciousness that we can daydream, make up lies, and write beautiful poems and scientific theories... Thus we might think of consciousness as intentionally ordered information... We may call intentions the force that keeps information in consciousness ordered. (p. 57)

Dr. Csikszentmihalyi's thesis on consciousness is important to ponder. The idea of consciousness as a clearinghouse suggests that we all have the potential to use consciousness to guide our actions. The question that lingers, however, is why do we not activate this clearinghouse perspective more often.

It seems that this question of consciousness focuses on two major dimensions, internal (me) and external (you). Although differences can be painful, they can also lead to the next logical action;

what can I do about this? As the different person's consciousness gets pushed and pulled, primarily through the pain of reality and rejection, a light can appear at the end of the tunnel. This light, the reality of change, presents both a formidable challenge and opportunity. The challenge lies with the painful internal and external review of the situation.

It is important to factor in the time that might lapse as our consciousness ponders the pain, confusion or frustration of difference. It could happen quickly or might linger for years. This time frame is highly variable and difficult to predict. I have friends who have turned around their difference quickly and others who still struggle.

2

Understanding Difference

It is the mark of the cultured man that he is aware of the fact that equality is an ethical and not a biological principle.

Ashley Montague

2

Understanding Difference

Before we can understand the broader aspects of difference, it is important to appreciate the standards which offset those things perceived as different. That is, things are only considered to be different if they deviate from what is perceived as typical.

It is also important to know that every element of the human experience has limits or parameters of acceptance and rejection. Consider human intelligence. Although suspect, we do have measures that offer some gauge to intelligence. These tests are routinely given and render scores that rate people. Administered over thousands of children of similar age, these test scores are divided at various cutoff levels. A high, low, and median are established and then individual scores are rated off these intervals. Children are then said to be slow, gifted, or average based on where they fall in test scores. The slow or gifted children are clearly perceived and then treated by the school district as different. Indeed, most of the offerings within the typical school curriculum are designed for the average student. This often forces the slow or gifted students out of the school district to special schools if they are going to grow in the educational experience.

This example offers two points for consideration. One is the establishment of dimensions to gauge normalcy, or the average. With standard IQ, the typical range for the average is between 70 and 130 in scores. These numbers represent the norm. Most people who are tested fall into this category. The other element of this example suggests that children who score outside the norm are better off in another school that caters to their "kind."

Another example might be found with a physical dimension such as height or weight. Indeed, we are all painfully aware of "acceptable" weight levels as we see them advertised and the weight loss centers display them all the time. If you fall in the norm, most of our societal amenities are geared for you. Seats, and doors, and cars, and most public spaces are designed for the average. If you are bigger, or smaller than the norm, you often have to get special fits or designs. These special fits can be costly, embarrassing, and stigmatic.

Thus, difference occurs when a person is found, or thought to be, outside of the norm. As mentioned earlier, regardless if the difference was self induced, caused by someone else, or unplanned, the perspectives of society remain much the same – that the person is different.

Consider these graphic examples that display deviancy and the norm.

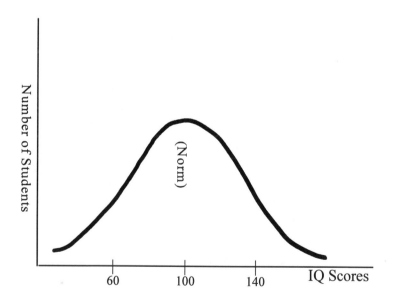

Distribution Curve of IQ Score

This issue of the norm is important. Statistically, sociologists can talk about the parameters of the norm, and as in the case of IQ, literally establish the boundaries. Yet, in actuality, these norms and their borders are highly variable and relevant. That is, what is considered the norm in one community for a particular issue, might be shifted and adjusted in another community. An example here might be the norm for homeowner upkeep. The standards set by one neighborhood might be very different from the standards of another. I've been in some communities where the standards are so different that they can appear deviant in and of themselves. One community I know will not allow people in the complex to work on their cars in their driveways. This may appear too working class for this upscale neighborhood, thus any auto work must be done in the garage. Where I come from, such a rule would be mocked.

Very few issues of human behavior and lifestyle are universal in standards. This is not to mean that all human behavior and lifestyle issues are always widely variant. Some are, others are not, but most have some variation in the standards imposed to define difference.

Indeed, even some items that may seem universal such as health, safety, or life and death issues can bring on debate. In some cultures, to die or to take a life may be considered heroic, whereas in another part of the world such an act would be a criminal penalty or theological sin.

This is a key point because it suggests that the parameters that have been established around a human behavior or lifestyle issue can be influenced or changed, even ones that are deeply rooted. It shows that determinants that can set people with difference apart, can be adjusted. It means that the reactions of society to difference are created by society, thus can be changed by society.

This notion of change, even to deeply held issues, is a vital one. When a critical mass of people start to change or shift in behavior, the standard can change. A simple example might be found in office dress style. There was a time when most business positions demanded dark suit, white shirt and tie. Over a period of time, dress style started to shift. Perhaps some people got away with wearing blue shirts with their dark suits. Whatever, a change started and the norms shifted. Today, dress styles can be widely variant. In fact, the ALCOA Corporation in Pittsburgh has regular casual days during the summer where employees can work in more relaxed apparel.

This thinking, however, pushes us to examine the concept of critical mass. In some situations, influential people in the community can start to push a culture or lifestyle change. Entertainers, athletes, and artists, indeed, any group in the public eye, can become trend setters that affect the norms of society. Things that might have been considered sacred in one era, are challenged and in many cases changed by those considered influential.

Still, it takes a following of people to push a change to be culturally accepted. To a certain extent, this is how a fad might be explained. A publicly recognized person introduces a change in appearance or dress. This leads to their followers starting to mimic the change. As the change moves further into the mainstream, it becomes socially sanctioned. In this process, it is hard to say exactly when the change becomes adopted as a mainstream action. Still, this is the basic flow of fashion or lifestyle change and it can happen with virtually anything.

This notion is critical when thinking about difference of people that is beyond their power to control or change. That is, a person who uses a wheelchair and is treated in stereotypical ways obviously may not be able to walk again, but might be able to influence a change in how people feel about them. In the context of this point on parameters of acceptance, it means that the most viable point for change is found with the attitudes of the community, not the different individual. There is no universal standard that says all people must walk or that people who use wheelchairs are not welcome.

CATEGORIES OF DIFFERENCE

When I think about difference and human behavior/lifestyle, three major categories come to mind. These categories and their review are:

PHYSICAL

The first major grouping of difference is physical. This means that the person who is different has a physical manifestation that is obvious and usually observable by others. This dimension includes people who are larger, or smaller than the norm. People we call giants or dwarfs. It also in- *little people* cludes people with less typical physical functioning. People who use wheelchairs or other mobility devices. It also relates to people who look different, due either to

> *The danger of overspecialization is that when the environment changes, you're stranded.*
>
> Sagan/Druyan

culture (turbans or veils) or accidental disfigurement (skin grafts from a severe facial burn). Additionally, it can include sensory difference such as sight, hearing or seizure situations. Indeed, any physical situation that renders a person different from what is perceived as the norm would fall into this category.

This physical category is the most obvious in this explanation of difference. Indeed, if one is considered different, they are almost automatically thought to have some physical manifestation. It is usually predictable that people's first thoughts when seeing or hearing the word "disabled" is that of wheelchairs.

COGNITIVE

The cognitive area deals with thinking, abstraction, memory, intelligence. Again, difference here would relate to any deviance in these areas either congenital or acquired. This category includes people with retardation, learning disabilities, memory or judgement issues caused by traumatic head injury, seizure disorder, geniuses or any other cognitive issue that pushes people outside the norm of what is considered or perceived as typical. This dimension also can apply to people who harbor thoughts or ideologies that are outside of the norm. Cults, fringe religious groups, and other associations that believe or subscribe to things that are not generally accepted or understood would fall in this category.

It is important to note here, that some people with cognitive difference are often not quickly detectable. It usually takes a few rounds of interchange before the difference is recognized. This subtleness can work to help the person "pass," but once the difference is detected the stigma can be deep.

EMOTIONAL

This final category deals with feelings and emotions. Although not always observable, emotional dimensions can influence behavior outside of the lines of acceptance. People who struggle with mental health issues (depression, schizophrenia, etc.), phobias, fears, and other concerns of the mind are often perceived as different and then treated accordingly. Again, consistent with this thesis, any emotional situation that was congenital or acquired and moves the person outside of the ascribed levels of acceptance would fall into this category.

> *The tendency to assume the worst about a given product may reflect some personal or institutional insecurity.*
>
> A. Kohn

As with the cognitive domain, the emotional area is difficult to initially detect. Once it is learned or observed, however, it takes a powerful hold and is extremely challenging to reverse. Often, the notion that a person is "crazy" can lead to strong social distantiation.

As basic as this review might seem, most situations of difference should fall into one of these three categories. Indeed, there are some severe situations of difference where a person might fall into a combination or even all three of these categories. For example, a person who has had a traumatic head injury might display, physical, cognitive, as well as emotional reactions to their accident. As one might expect, a combination of difference adds to the challenge and can create even greater difficulties.

Often, it is these more awesome experiences of difference that push our awareness. They tend to be more overt and sensational, thus observable. Yet difference, and the effects of difference abound. There is nary a one of us who have not been in a difference role at some point in our lives.

REACTIONS TO DIFFERENCE

Anyone who has experienced an obvious difference knows that there are two major reactions that typically follow; internal and external dynamics. Although the manifestations can happen to greater or lesser degrees, these internal and external reactions swirl in and around the different person. That is, when someone is different, they are often treated in negative and rejective ways. These external hostilities create a tone and then often lead to internal feelings of weakness and inability. These reactions are strongly associated and need to be examined separately.

EXTERNAL REACTIONS

The most obvious reactions are of ignorance, fear, and rejection. Quite simply, the different person is often not understood. Since they are not within the acceptable parameters, the typical lay person might be ignorant of the conditions that have precipitated the difference. This ignorance can then lead to a fear or misunderstanding of the difference. Indeed, some sociologists have articulated that the most common reaction to difference is caution and fear among adults. Interestingly enough, this fear is probably a conditioned reflex. That is, seeing difference sets into play a natural curiosity, but inquiries into the difference can lead to issues of fear. This is then usually ingested into a reactive behavior. Usually children show an innocent curiosity, but by adulthood most people become suspicious and fearful.

I am constantly amazed at the openness children show to difference. Recently, a friend from Canada came to visit me to compare some ideas about difference and inclusion. Along with his academic interest in this topic he also had some first hand experience. When he was a teenager he lost both arms in a sledding accident. Now he uses two hooks for arms, and when he visited we were right in the middle of a family gathering on "Condeluci Hill." As I introduced Jeff around to my family, the adults were somewhat unnerved by his hooks, but the children were incredibly interested. They wanted to know how he made them work, how he could pick up a hot dog, but more amazingly, how he maneuvered the mustard jar to embellish it.

Given all this, somewhere and someway, this innocence of childhood gives way to adult caution, and then to some type of distantiation. I am sure that we have some primal signals that kick in when we encounter difference, I'm just not sure if they are the ones of caution. In fact, some theorists suggest that we have a very basic empathy instinct that may somehow get corrupted as we age. One study, done through the National Institute of Health, found an empathy factor with infants and toddlers put in social situations. Most maternity ward nurses will testify that often when one infant cries, they all start to cry. Could this be coincidence or does the crying stir some basic form of empathy with infants?

It is also interesting to note that another feeling or assumption, usually associated with caution and fear, is a sense that the different person is responsible for their situation. This responsibility aspect is then followed by a second assumption that the different person is bad, evil or inept to have allowed the difference to occur. An example might be the belief that God is punishing the person who is different because they deserve to be punished. We have all heard people say, "they probably got what they deserve." Or, "they made their own bed, now they have to lie in it."

The combination of ignorance and fear then blend to cause a variety of actions that are shunning in nature. This rejection can be openly hostile and aggressive where people are mistreated or actively scorned. Indeed, historical perspectives that look at deviance have shown that different people have been beaten, imprisoned, ostracized, or outwardly destroyed. Wolfensberger's exposé on deviance and deathmaking offers example after example of the ways people who are different through disability are offset, victimized, or destroyed (1987).

There are other, less overt ways that different people are rejected. In today's society, the best example of this softer version of rejection is discrimination. There is hardly a person reading this book who does not know the rejecting nature of discrimination. If it has not happened directly to you, surely you know someone who has experienced this modern-day version of exclusion.

Discrimination exists in all walks of life, from housing to jobs to lifestyle opportunities. Although it has been most publicly articulated in racial dimensions, it is experienced with most types of difference. The mother of young children who is not promoted in her job because she seems to be more committed to family; the person with a disability who is not hired; the black person who is treated in suspicious ways by the sales clerk in an exclusive department store, are all examples of discrimination. Indeed, it is difference, and the fear or misunderstanding of difference that is the mother of discrimination. No person who has a difference is free from the ugliness of this form of rejection.

And so, external reactions to difference abound. Regardless of the type of difference, physical, cognitive or emotional, people who fall into any (or all) of these categories are vulnerable to the ignorance, fear and rejection. These reactions, however, are so powerful and sweeping that people with difference are clearly affected in how they feel about themselves. This leads to the next reaction.

INTERNAL REACTIONS

There is a sociological concept that was covered earlier in this text that relates to role expectation and role behavior. Simply stated, when people are cast into certain roles in deep and pervasive ways, usually the expectations that surround the role lead to the antici-pated behavior. That is, when the expectations and standards sur-rounding an individual are clear and precise, the behavior will usu-ally follow. As was mentioned earlier, this is true in positive as well as negative examples.

Thus, as people with some sort of difference hear, feel, and see the external reactions of ignorance, fear and rejection, it is predict-able that these reactions will have a strong cutting effect on their behavior. The result is an assault on self-confidence and self-esteem. How could it not be, when the predominant reaction to the differ-ent person is a negative and rejective one?

It is vital to note here, the importance, and, to a point, the vulnerability of self-esteem. How one feels about oneself creates a deep tone for how one acts and reacts to situations. This notion of self-esteem has been examined in many works, but one report I found to be of particular use in understanding self-esteem and dif-ference is the California Task Force Report on Self-Esteem (1990). This review presents an articulate explanation of how self-esteem is often damaged by societies reaction to difference, and how we con-tinue to judge people in comparison to some "Madison Avenue" norm.

Of course, as confidence and esteem are eroded, one's dignity is on the line. It's hard to be dignified when you are feared or rejected. As this occurs then, energy, motivation and willingness give way to isolation and seclusion. Quite simply, it becomes a survival mecha-nism to steer clear of the assaults. To venture out is to be reminded of one's difference and rejection. It becomes easier to stay with one's "own kind."

Consequently, people of difference might retreat to a place where they are safe, and to a certain extent, accepted and respected. In many regards, this sanctuary is essential to one's mental health. The pangs of difference and rejection are just too intense.

This action, however, is misunderstood by society. Rather than seeing the cycle of deviance, and its role in offsetting people, most lay people just assume "that they would rather be together." Or, that they are better off with "their own kind." Thus, the cycle is perpetuated and hardened. Stereotypes are confirmed, and then passed on to others and the script intensifies.

3

The Dualistic Society

*Our relations with
one another are
ultimately rooted in
what we are.*

Ram Dass

The Dualistic Society

To a certain extent, the external and internal reactions lead way to a dualistic society. One, for those in the "norm," the other, for those who are different. This is not only hurtful to people with difference, but it is harmful to society. It is harmful because a society defines itself through its diversity, not similarity. It is the differences of life that truly create an enrichment to our culture and society. So dualism hurts everyone.

I best understand, this notion of the importance of diversity, through my family roots and current situation. In 1917, when my dad's family came to America from Italy, they moved to McKees Rocks, PA (a suburb of Pittsburgh) and rented a home on a hillside in the Italian section of the community. As the family grew, my dad and his eight brothers and sisters would play regularly up on the hill above their home. Indeed, my grandfather kept his goats and tomato patch on the hill, keeping a watchful eye on his crops and his children.

After World War II, my dad and Uncle Sam decided to buy the hill that had been so important to them as children. With a handshake deal they bought the land and started to move up. First, a home for Uncle Sam, then my dad, and then their dad. What followed was a humble compound that today houses some 15 Condeluci families. It is truly a safe and distinct place.

As I grew up on "Condeluci Hill," I had a wonderful sense of security and acceptance, a feeling that continues today. I know that whatever happens to me, I will be loved and welcomed on the hill. This is a vital feeling of protection, yet if I do not venture off the hill, my growth will be stunted. That is, I know I am on safe the hill, but I only learn *who* I am when I meet different people. This comparison helps me place myself in the larger scheme of community and brings a true enrichment. The singular experience of the hill, although it is important to my security and initial self-worth, is merely a starting point for life. It is the diversity, however, that brings the true spice.

People need other people. They need them to feel love and security. They also need others to discover who they are and to find a course in which to grow. Quite simply, diversity leads to growth.

Yet, to a large extent, our society has become a dualistic haven. One for us and the other for them, whoever them may be. If you think about your own community in terms of groups, you can easily identify them. They are the elderly off in some high-rise, or the poor off in some ghetto, or the people with disabilities off in some group home, or the wealthy off in some country club, or the sick off in some hospital.

Now, if you contemplate these groupings you find that some are chosen, even aspired to; some are self-imposed and others are chosen for people. To some extent, these groupings may not be bad. In fact, some might argue that for a group such as the sick, the clustering in hospitals might be good.

For me, as I think about dualism and grouping, I don't necessarily see evil. Some good can come to people who band together for common cause. I do however, get concerned when groups of people are relegated to a setting because another group of people feel it is "best" for them. This concept gets hardened when the relegated group has no recourse, alternative or options in the process. If the grouping is seen as important for clinical or therapeutic reasons, then it becomes virtually impenetrable.

When I share these thoughts in public forums, there is always a pundit who challenges me with stark examples such as prisons for those who have done wrongs against society. Surely, these people must be kept apart. Now I'm not about suggesting total inclusion to the point of fanaticism. In some cases, there are times and places where people perhaps ought to be relegated and, maybe prisons fall here. What concerns me, however, is when the relegation becomes common place and the group being offset has no say in the matter. Our society is filled with example after example of these types of situations.

So what are we to do? How do we best move to address difference? What type of services, supports or understanding are necessary to carve a more welcoming society; one that is more open and receptive? Before we try to answer these questions, we need to examine how our current society attempts to deal with difference.

Dealing With Difference

Although we know that in an informal sense, the way society deals with difference is to reject, avoid or banish the different person, some in society have attempted to reach out and support different people. Over the years, these efforts have formalized and today we call these more structured actions human or domestic services. These are the various programs for groups such as the sick, disabled or poor in our communities. They include projects for the elderly, or vulnerable children, or the mentally retarded. They take all kinds of shape and form and emanate from both public and private sources.

> Civilized men have gained notable mastery over energy, matter, and inanimate nature generally...but, by contrast, we appear to be living in the Stone Age so far as our handling of human relationships in concerned.
>
> G. Allport

In the United States, these activities have their roots with the British Poor Laws. They have, over time, taken on a fiercely American character, but still anchor with the thoughts that a civilized society takes care of its different, who are often thought to be sick or poor.

In the United States, Canada, and other northern European societies these formal efforts to look after the different become a strong objective of the government. There seems to be a more social agenda present for those who are different. Regardless of emanation, most formal or structured approaches to difference in industrialized nations is to do typically one (or all) of three things. Let's explore each separately. These are:

1. To fix the difference
2. To maintain the different person
3. To change the broader understanding about the difference

FIXING THE DIFFERENCE

Since most difference is considered to be aberrant or negative, it is natural to find the fixing approach to be the major way we deal with difference. It is important to recognize that the "fix them" approach emanates from a medical model. In this approach, the difference is seen as a deficiency and the expert rushes in to apply a treatment plan. In my book *Interdependence*, I examined the detail and emphasis of the medical model. Clearly, the dominance of the medical model has had a primary emphasis on changing or fixing the difference. It is an effort to make the person whole again and to fit into the norm.

Given this common approach of trying to fix that which we consider different, consider these situations:

A person is poor – Let's fix them to have job skills.
A person is not well – Let's fix them to be better.
A person has a speech impediment – Let's fix them so they can talk better.
A person is depressed – Let's fix them to be able to better cope.

A child does not make the team – Let's fix him to have
more skills to better compete.
A student is not so bright – Let's fix them to know more.
And on, and on, and on.

Now with these examples come two thrusts; one is that the
person can be fixed to do something. This means that the attention
is on truly changing the person – a highly microscopic activity. The
other is that the person, through some adjustment to their person,
can be fixed to fit in as best as possible. An example here might be
when a person learns something or uses some device or equipment
to lessen the effects of difference – still a highly microscopic activity.

I say microscopic, because with both thrusts (the person changes,
or something is added to the person), the onus is specific to the
different person; they must make the adjustment. It is all up to the
different person, and if they do not or cannot make the change,
they are usually positioned as the failure.

To understand all this, one only need visit a local program designed for people who have some difference. Take a job preparation
program for someone who is unemployed for example; in this setting you will find people who are jobless working on a number of
techniques all designed to help (or fix) them so they can get a job or
better compete in the job market. They might be learning a new
skill, or enhancing an existing skill, or being coached on how to
develop a resume, or be role playing a mock interview.

I recently visited a friend who works for a local shelter and soup
kitchen. As I spent time helping out, I was struck by two major
things. One was the number of families at the kitchen to take meals.
The typical stereotype of hunger and homelessness usually doesn't
include families. The other point of impact for me was the number
of fix'em programs the shelter also provided. There were classes,
and job attainment activities and a number of other things happening to help fix these hungry and often homeless people.

All of these kind of activities are microscopic. They mandate
that the jobless person change something about them to move out

of this area of difference, or that the homeless person change something about them to help them out of their plight.

Another example might be a center for people with retardation. Again, we would find a number of people with the similarity of retardation kept together to teach them new things. They might be learning how to read basic menus, or community signs, or they might be practicing how to act more appropriate or typical when out in public. Most programs for people with disabilities follow this format.

I remember an experience I had not so long ago, when I went to visit a friend who works at a sheltered workshop. I arrived before the workers had gotten their assignments and I found my friend, Jim, sitting in a large holding area with many other "clients" of this program. I sat with Jim and we began talking. Soon, the foreman entered the room and began calling out people's names. I sat with Jim until he was called and then we both walked to the place of his assignment. Since the foreman didn't know me, he pause as I walked by, but my clear intent to follow Jim made him think I was just another "client" called to assignment. We arrived at Jim's station and he explained to me the nature of his work. He was to do a small task in assembling bicycle brakes. After the brakes were assembled, another crew took them apart. A third crew served as "runners" to shuttle the assembled and disassembled parts back and forth. Finally, a fourth crew went to classes to learn how to be "appropriate" in the work setting. Even though I have worked in human services for people with disabilities for some 24 years, this experience with Jim really drove home the senselessness of many of our so called "programs."

In all of these examples, people are working to get ready to participate or engage so as to lose the impact of their difference. That is, if the poor person gets a job, they have made great strides toward eradicating their difference, or if the retarded person can now perform some function in a more community accepted way, the effects of their retardation will be lessened. They will become more like you and me – the great community norm.

As we think about this propensity to fix these different people it is important to know that the fixer, the person in control are usually the ones to judge success or failure. Indeed, some standard or measure, again initiated by the fixer, is the gauge used to deem outcome. This means that usually the different person has very little to say about not only what they are doing, but how they are doing other than to parrot the standard established by the fixer.

THE "FIX THEM" SCRIPT

To better appreciate these ways of dealing with difference, we can look at a number of different tongue-in-cheek scripts. The first is a fix'em script that goes something like this:

> We have deemed you to be identified as different, and as such we feel you should be fixed. Therefore, we know the best place for you, it's a place we typicals have developed for you. Here, you can be with your own, be exposed to what you need to change in order to be with us. You must work hard, however, if you want to alleviate your difference. We'll tell you how you are doing, and we will deem when you have made it. At that time, you are free to take your fixed self out there and mix it up. If something goes wrong, however, don't blame us. After all, it's you who are different.

MAINTAINING, OR TO BE WITH YOUR OWN

This next thrust of dealing with difference pushes beyond the "fix them" programs for people who have just not made it.

At this level, in many situations, the different person has been worked with or on, and still is not capable of change. Maybe they don't want to, or maybe they just can't. Rather than giving up on the person and sending them away the energy of the system turns to maintenance. This often translates into a low budget effort to watch over them.

An example here might be found in a school system where students are having some problems learning assignment. The "fix them" approach would first offer some remedial classes to try to catch them up. Maybe some equipment like computers or calculators will be introduced to push learning.

When it becomes clear that these different students will not or cannot learn, a maintenance approach will begin. That is, the "slow" students will all be kept together and either entertained, or just tolerated until the time frames run out. At this point, little or no resources or energy will be utilized. In the scheme of things, extras for this group are just not worth it.

This example of the maintenance of students is exceptionally relevant for me. I remember a specific class I had as a high school student that fit this mold to a tee. Since I was in a group considered to be lower level students, the only standard established by the faculty member who handled the study hall was for us to not kill ourselves or others. I remember him saying, "Just don't make any noise, you can sleep, draw, read comic books, anything, but keep yourself and me out of trouble."

Another example of maintenance might be found at the senior citizens center. If there is little that can be taught to the elderly, the center will find a comfortable way to just take care of them. A visit to any neighborhood senior citizen center will display some people who fit the "maintain 'em" mold.

"Maintenance" Script

At this level the script goes something like this:

We typical people who care have done all we can to fix you; obviously you are unfixable. We can't be terrible to admit this and send you out into the night, so instead we will keep you here with your own kind. It is better for you and you know how much we care. Now, be a good sport and sit quietly in you chair, we'll let you know when you can leave.

SINCE WE CAN'T CHANGE YOU, WE'LL CHANGE THE WORLD

In this third approach, formal services for people with difference turn some attention to macroscopics. That is, either along with fixing the different persons, or maintaining them, some energy is also applied to helping the world understand "them."

Surely, you are aware of the myriad of associations and organizations dedicated to helping the world understand their particular cause. As you think about this, count up the ones interested in you knowing about their form of difference. A simple turn to the phone book "blue pages" should do the trick. Here, you will find everything you wanted to know about difference, but were afraid to ask.

In this category, you might find the support group who wants you to know about myasthenia gravis (or pick any other diagnosis). They have brochures, pamphlets, speakers bureau, newsletter, information hot line, public service announcements, celebrity spokesperson, and the like, all working to enhance your knowledge and understanding of the malady. They testify before Congress, city hall, church groups, school assemblies, or any other forum who is willing to listen.

Ignorance is less remote from truth than prejudice.

D. Diderot

Often, their stories are filled with the ravages of the difference, how the afflicted have suffered, how society has misjudged and how the listener can make a difference. Usually, this last point means give money. To get good, thorough attention, the horror stories are amplified.

It is interesting what gets people's attention, and then what they remember from the encounter. Usually, it is the drama and intensity of the story. We tend to remember the sensational, and so that is what these groups do – sensationalize the difference. Not all of them, but more than most do.

"UNDERSTAND THEM" SCRIPT

The script for this group like this:

Listen to us fellow community member, we need to tell you about this problem (difference) that some people have. It is a terrible problem, and no one in their right mind would want to have it – but some do, and we can't turn our backs. Can't you see it clear to give some money (time, attention, service, understanding, sympathy, pity, clothes, other hand-outs) so we can make life better for "them."

As you ruminate on these three scripts, recognize that they all emanate from a we/they point of view. They all utilize experts or spokespersons and are downward in the way they play out — with the different person on the down side of the equation.

FEATURES COMMONLY ASSOCIATED WITH DIFFERENCE

Now, with all three ways of dealing with difference, there are some common threads that are worthy of time and attention here. They are found in every circumstance just discussed, and after a closer look, they are important to stigma and perpetuation of the difference. These are:

COMMON IDENTIFICATION

Label jars not people

Obviously, a common identification or label is the start point for all formal treatment of difference. That is, some common trait is usually identified to unify the difference. This might come in the form of a diagnosis or medical opinion. Various disabilities and diseases would fall into this category. Or there might be a social context for the difference, such as poverty, or being an "at risk" group such as homosexual or drug user. Whatever, some type of common identity always precedes the initiation of a formal service.

NEGATIVE OR DEFICIT PERSPECTIVE

wanting/needy

Attached to the common identification, is that most difference at the point of formal actions or service is usually looked at from a negative or needs perspective. By this, I mean that the commonality of the difference is often set apart by what wrong is caused by the difference. This is evident when you think about the typical features of most labels of difference. With AIDS for example, the common understanding is immune breakdown and ultimately death. With aging, you have the impact of chronic deterioration of the body. With learning disabilities, you have the difficulty in cognitive processing of information. And on and on. Hardly a difference is detached from its negative or deficit features.

CONGREGATION

grouping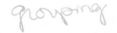

Another common factor is the congregation and, in some cases, the isolation of the different group. Most formal services, be they "fix 'em," "maintain 'em," or "tell 'em," bring all the different people together at some points. This might be for some service or for mutual support.

This congregation or grouping is thought to be natural, as if the different people are happier, or better off with their own kind.

Further, it is felt that they can be better taught, served, treated, or maintained when they are grouped.

ROLE OF HELPER OR EXPERT

With most formal approaches to difference, some helper or expert is present. Often, their role is to lead, guide, teach, assess, represent, or maintain the different person. It is also safe to assume that the helper or expert does not possess or currently have the difference of their congregation. That is to say, if the reason for the difference is homelessness, it is probably safe to assume that the expert in charge of the homeless shelter has a home. Or that the director of the UCP center does not have cerebral palsy. Or that the director of the senior citizen center is usually not a senior.

These themes undergird most formal approaches to difference. They are so prominent and insidious that we hardly think of them. They are business as usual with agencies and organizations that surround people who have some type of difference and at first glance, are seemingly innocent. Yet, when explained in a more detail these approaches to difference can, in fact, be destructive rather than helpful.

To put this in perspective, we need to set the tone for not only the effects of difference, but the effects of formal approaches to difference. Let's first turn to the general effects of difference.

EFFECTS OF DIFFERENCE

When people's difference becomes known to the culture, I believe certain effects play out between the different person and society at large. In fact, these effects can occur even if a formal agency or organization is working to address the difference. These effects follow a graded format and cascade from a perspectives of least distantiating to most. They are:

Effects of Difference
Destroyed
Banished
Banned
Excluded
Not Welcomed
Avoided
Misunderstood

MISUNDERSTOOD

The most relaxed effect of difference is to be misunderstood. Many of us can relate to this feeling, as at some point in our lives, we have experienced being misunderstood. This may have happened when you felt yourself to be the only person who seems to understand or appreciate a situation. To be misunderstood is to be queer, or strange or odd, but still basically respected. At this

> *Tolerance is the positive and cordial effort to understand another's beliefs, practices, and habits without necessarily sharing or accepting them.*
> *J. Liebman*

level, people shake their heads at your behavior, and sometimes talk behind your back, but you still fit into the system. An important awareness, however, is that the misunderstood person starts to doubt or question themselves. Being misunderstood can begin to erode one's self concept.

I'm sure you know people who fall into this category. I have a friend who is always at the fringe of a circle of people I know. Although he is invited to gatherings he just doesn't connect with the group. Often, I'm the primary link he has with this particular circle. I am certain he is not long for our group.

Know that misunderstanding can happen for a variety of reasons. At times, if someone's lifestyle changes, the effects can play out in behaviors, appearances, or actions. These changes can bring episodes of misunderstanding from friends or associates who are used to the "old" patterns. As with other points explored in this text, the changes in behavior could affect physical or cognitive issues and could have internal or external implications. That is, if a person begins to embrace ideas or thoughts that extend outside their circle, this shift can make the individual feel different from their network. The change might manifest in physical actions and these new behaviors then place the person at risk of misunderstanding.

An example here might be a person who begins to think differently about a topic such as church. I know a woman who began to question her family religion and as her thoughts evolved she felt the need to challenge her traditional religious beliefs. After a period of time, she found that she needed to leave the church and begin a new form of worship. In the process of the shift, she told me how misunderstood she felt by family members who could just not understand her reasons. The stage of misunderstandings is truly an awkward one.

AVOIDED

The next step, after being misunderstood, is to be avoided. This is when people clearly start to move away from you as your oddity becomes less of a quirk, and more of a representation of your personality. To be avoided is to have people look away, or to acknowledge others instead of you. At this level you can still be present, but eyes don't meet, and hospitality is clearly checked.

A good example of this stage was illustrated in the movie, "The Way We Were," with Barbara Streisand and Robert Redford. In this film, the two main characters are drawn together, yet very different in backgrounds and beliefs. Initially, the Streisand character is misunderstood by Redford's circle. Then, as she continues to hold firm to her convictions, she is avoided by members of the circle.

Avoidance is a sanctioned form of distantiation. All of us have had experiences where we have moved to avoid a person we know or might even respect because we feel uncomfortable having an exchange. Some people avoid others because they feel inadequate or inept in social settings. Others avoid exchange because they don't like what an other might believe or express.

In any example, avoidance suggests that both parties have a right to be present, only that they don't want to exchange. This right to presence offers a level of equality among players. Even though they may be very different from each other, this level summons at least the chance that people might interact.

NOT WELCOMED

As difference drives a deeper wedge, the next effect is the first basic step of rejection, that of not being welcomed. At this level, you clearly feel the pangs of distantiation. You know you are not welcomed because all the signs reinforce your oddity. Your difference becomes a clear issue that sets you apart. By this stage, your personal feelings of inadequacy are clear and distinct. You are different and not welcomed.

Earlier in this work, I told a story about the time, while attending a national conference, I was invited to sit in caucus with a group of folks, all who had disabilities. For many of those present, I was clearly not welcomed. Although I had a bridge to the group, the majority in the circle did not want me present. I was just not welcomed.

A typical manifestation of not being welcomed is found in either overt or indirect messages that signal a displeasure at your presence. These signs could be glances, eye contact or stares, or subtle mumbling between people that you know is about you. In more direct ways, people will walk away or will find a more formal way to escort you out.

My dad has told me stories of his boyhood; a time when immigrants were not always easily embraced. After graduation from high school he got a job at the steel mill in Pittsburgh. He wanted to fit in and one day made his way to a tavern frequented by other workers. He quickly learned, however, that Italians were not welcomed in this tavern as he was not just asked to leave, but physically escorted to the door. It was a powerful message at a tender age.

EXCLUDED

At this stage, the difference is clearly distinguished and the different person is blatantly excluded from the mainstream. All signals reinforce that your presence is not only not welcomed, but you have been consciously excluded from actions of the group. In some cases, architecture excludes people with disabilities, or admission charges exclude people of poverty, or language excludes people who are illiterate. Ask anyone who is considered, or perceives themselves as different about the signs of exclusion and they will tell you example after example.

In some cases, exclusion (or some of the other identified effects) might not be consciously intended or malicious by design, but the effect is just as prominent. When people are not included, for whatever reason, it is a strong and often painful feeling. It says loud and clear – we don't want you with our kind.

I have been intrigued by a growing polarization that now lingers between being excluded and banned, that relates to smoking in our society. Clearly today, smokers are devalued. They have been excluded from many places and are now banned in most public places. I personally have become aware of this exclusion of smokers, as I don't see friends of mine, who are smokers, as much. It's as if this one type of behavior, smoking, has now become the key point of difference between me and others who smoke. I noticed, at a recent party, that no smokers were present. I then began to think of the smokers I know from the larger circle of this group and it was stark to me that the smokers of this larger group had been consciously excluded at this gathering.

Now this situation of smoking raises an interesting variable–that of safe and unsafe elements of difference. With all the evidence of the dangerous effects of second-hand smoke, the exclusion of smokers from the group can be justified by those who exclude for safety precautions. In fact, people have created many a reason (excuse) to historically exclude people. Many groups of people have been kept apart because it was felt that their mere presence was (or is) a threat to the community.

BANNED

By this level, the exclusion has become formalized. That is, specific laws, rules, and regulations literally legalize, or attempt to legitimize the distantiation through a banning. Often, these laws, rules, and regulations are illegal, or at least immoral, nonetheless are usually accepted or sanctioned by the mainstream.

From time to time, I have done some work in Galveston, Texas, and once during a visit, a friend who grew up on the island took me to the public library. This beautiful stone building was erected at the turn of the century, a wonderful time for architecture. Unfortunately, it was not such a wonderful time for a group of Americans who were virtually banned from a variety of public buildings. There on this magnificent building, etched in stone for future generations to understand, was the lettering, "No Coloreds." A loud and direct manifestation of banning a different group, caught for future generations to carry out.

Banning exists today in all types of ways. From the signs in the window "No T-shirts" to the rules and regulations of club memberships, some people, for whatever legitimate reasons, are edited out of the exchange.

BANISHED

Although this is an operationalization of being banned, the concept of banishment is a tad more intense. To be banned from certain buildings or services is one thing, but to be banished from a community, society, or civilization is the ultimate punishment. Indeed, the most lethal of punishment is taking one's life, or capital punishment, but some criminologists contend that banishment is more penalizing than death. Imagine being alive, but not being allowed to meet, talk or associate with others. Some suggest that this is a fate worse than death.

Another distinction between banishment and being banned is that with banning, there is a flicker of hope that the ban might be lifted. Banishment, on the other hand, offers no such chance. It is a much more permanent phenomena.

DESTRUCTION

The final effect of difference is the ultimate one, death. History is riddled with examples of ways and means that people of difference have been categorically eliminated by those who were valued. The most prominent example, of course, is Nazi Germany and the plight of the Jews. Here was a generation of people whose difference, their religion, set the stage for their destruction at the hands of the Aryans. It is interesting to note that in Nazi Germany, well before the extermination of the Jews, people with disabilities and retardation were eliminated in an effort to perfect the Aryan means of destruction. One researcher discovered that in the early years of the war, the Germans, under Hitler's orders, bombed a number of their own hospitals and sanitariums that housed people with disabilities, mental illness and mental retardation. Then they calmly blamed these bombings on the English.

During a recent visit to the U.S. Holocaust Museum in Washington, D.C., all of these aforementioned effects of difference could be followed in relationship to Nazi Germany. In the 20s and early 30s, the effects of an economic recession on Germany caused Jews, as moneylenders to be misunderstood. In the early stages of rising anti-semitism, the Jews were first avoided and then not welcomed. Next, as the hatred became more formalized the Jews were then labeled so as to hasten their exclusion by having to wear a yellow Star of David on their clothes. Next, came the banning from various places and sections of town, then the banishment to the ghettos and then finally the destruction at the death camps. As I toured this museum, these stages unfolded in a horrible cascade.

It is interesting to note that as overt as destruction seems on the surface, there are many subtle elements to this phenomena. Some contend that abortion fits squarely into this discussion. Now I know abortion is an emotional topic with equal passions on both sides of the argument, but I had an experience that called the question of difference-related destruction. It happened a few years back when my wife was pregnant with our third child (Santino, for those of you who heard my talks or seen my slides). Since both of us were over 40 at the time, Liz's obstetrician suggested that we meet with the genetic counselors to talk about the pregnancy and our options. I remember sitting in an office at MacGee-Womens Hospital in Pittsburgh as the genetic counselor told us all about pregnancy past age 40, possible risks to the fetus and options for amniocentesis therapy to give us a clear picture of the developing baby. As we talked further she told us that there was a slight risk of miscarriage when the tests are done, but once the results are in you can be assured the baby is "healthy" (As if disability or Down's syndrome is unhealthy). She went on to say that if indeed there was evidence of a chromosome discrepancy we could decide to end the pregnancy. When she finished the explanation, I couldn't help but to be sadden by the point she was making – a family expecting a child with a disability might be better off if the child was aborted!. This area of destruction is one that still happens today.

And so, the effects of difference can ebb, flow, and range through a variety of actions. The net result in this crescendo, however, is an increasing absence of hospitality toward people perceived as different, and for most of us reading these words, at one time or another, we have felt some of these effects.

Know, however, that not all people who are different are subjected to negative consequences. Some groups are considered to be positively attractive. With geniuses, for example, it is interesting to note that they have their own separate group called MENSA. This is an exclusive club that only allows membership if you can pass a test and prove your intellectual superiority. Again, we see how difference can lead to a grouping and an offset experience, even if the difference is perceived to be positive.

The same elevation of esteem is true for people who have athletic or technical skill levels that push them outside the norm. These people too, are different, yet may be valued and respected. Indeed, today, to be an elite athlete is to open the doors to acknowledgment, stardom and incredible material rewards. In most cases, rather than people moving away from this type of difference, some strive to get as close as possible.

The same can be said for highly valued people who then take on a negatively ascribed difference through an accident or illness. In these cases, the power status from the positive pre-difference situation can often override the negative effects of the newly imposed difference. That is, if one encounters an experience that now makes that person different, those around the person tend to keep them in their pre-difference status level. If an actor or athlete experiences a disability that leads to the need for a wheelchair, the perspectives of how the person "used to be" can hold tight. This could be true even if the difference manifests the same as for typical people who may be avoided or socially banned in the same situation.

The only snag in this scenario is if the previously esteemed person receives that difference through behaviors that are thought to be inappropriate or immoral. In these cases, the behavior that led way to the difference overrides the previous esteem experienced by the person. An example here might be an actor or athlete who contracts AIDS through drug use. This negative action that created the difference; drug use for example, carries more weight than the pre-difference role and the person may be treated in negative ways.

This ability for people with difference to overcome the typical stigmas that follow is precisely why various groups that represent people with difference like to find, and then enlist, prominent people who have the difference as their spokes-people. Actors with AIDS, or athletes with epilepsy, or corporate leaders who have a family member with retardation all then become key links that attempt to push the negatives typically associated with the difference to a positive perspective.

This reality, however, of these prominent people who can still hold positive places in spite of their difference is an important notion indeed. It suggests that there is not some inbred element that creates the negative effects of difference. If a person on the street can accept a previously valued person from a typically devalued group, then too, they can accept anyone from that group. It affirms the notion that people in society create or determine what is considered different, and more importantly, who is considered different. If this is so, then society can equally adjust, augment or change its perspective. If we create the reaction to deviance, and that reaction is usually to offset, then we can change this same behavior to one that is welcoming. We are the masters of our collective destiny.

Albert Ellis (1975), the eminent psychologist, knows this phenomena well. In his work, he has developed a form of therapy called Rational Emotive Therapy (RET). In his thesis, if people are struggling with a psychological challenge, they can literally practice a rational approach to change. An example Ellis once used in a talk I attended, helped me understand RET. He asked us to consider the following scenario:

> You're on a crowded bus on your way home from a harrowing day. The bus is packed and you have to stand. Holding your brief case and a package, added to how tired you are from the day, you're not a particularly happy camper. The bus starts and stops and you are being jarred around. Then

you feel a piercing elbow to your back – someone has bumped into you trying to make their way to the front of the bus. You're highly annoyed and turn to give this person a piece of your mind. Then you notice their white cane. It's a person with a visual disability making their way up front. Automatically, your anger turns to compassion and you help forge an opening for the person to pass by.

In this example, Ellis suggests that the powerful emotional reaction of anger can quickly shift to compassion because your rationalization of the incident shifted from inconsiderate person to individual with a disability. The rational helps shift the emotion and then the behavior becomes very different.

I think this notion of RET has some relevance to the points made previously about people of prominence who have, or are seen with people who have a stigmatic situation. The rational is that if the prominent person, one who is respected and admired, is able to get beyond the stigma of difference, then the difference must not be that bad. The obvious next thought is that if they can alter their behavior toward the difference, so too can I.

4

How and When
Difference Occurs

*I have found power in the
mysteries of thought, exaltation
in the chanting of the Muses;
I have been versed in the rea-
sonings of men;
but fate is stronger than anything I have known.*

Euripides

How and When
Difference Occurs

As we continue to examine this phenomena of difference, another key element is found in looking at how difference occurs. Now, this notion, although seemingly simple, must be considered from an understanding of normative analysis. You might recall from an earlier section, that difference is a relative subject. Clearly, some people make a bigger deal of difference than others. Thus, in exploring how difference occurs we must factor in when difference might be commonly accepted. This means that although the difference may fall outside of the typical normative scale, people in general might not perceive the difference from a negative perspective. The earlier example we made of this phenomena was a genius, who scores different from the norm in IQ. Although they are deviant, they are usually not seen from a negative lens.

In another possibility, if a person feels some pangs of difference, even if the difference they perceive is within some limits of typical, this type of difference may not be outwardly negative. For example, if an adolescent is going through a period of acne, and feels very self conscious and different, this type of difference might be perceived by those around the person as somewhat typical to a person of their age. This is not to deny the pressure and anxiety that might be felt by the person with acne; only to acknowledge that to others the difference may not be significant.

Keeping this in mind, if a person experiences a type of societally sanctioned difference, the impact of the difference is lessened. If you stop and reflect, a number of socially sanctioned differences can be identified. Some are:

+ Voice change with maturity
+ Mood swings with menopause
+ Loss of hair in aging
+ Need for bifocals at middle age

In these examples, the person at the apex of these differences might feel awkward and uncomfortable, yet those around them may feel their difference is socially acceptable. This is particularly true of stages associated with natural development.

If, however, the difference is not sanctioned by society, the stigmatic residue will be stronger. That is, if a family has a child with a severe disability, this type of difference may fall outside of the boundaries of acceptance. Thus, to them, an element of distantiation will occur.

I know many such families who have children with severe disabilities and face a deep societal stigma that suggests there is something wrong with them. Somehow, someway they are led to feel a responsibility or blame for the difference that has befell their family. This phenomena can play out in strong ways. Some families feel ashamed, as if they are being punished for some wrong. This fits a script that people get what they deserve. Other families feel awkward, not knowing how to describe or define their situation. I know one family that continually kept apologizing for the situation of their child who had cerebral palsy.

In other situations, where a difference is thrust upon a family, such as in those surrounding an accident, a similar type of phenomena might occur. There might be outward signs, or inward feelings that the family did not serve as good parents. These themes suggest that the family is unsafe and could have prevented the accident or illness from occurring.

In both of these examples, the congenital or traumatic initiation of difference, the question of why us, or for the observer, why them, is present. We often have this sense that when bad things happen to people, they somehow deserved it.

This is a crazy, anchoring notion that can hold individuals or families hostage. Still, it plagues many a person or family. Indeed, Rabbi Harold Kushner (1982) has left his indelible mark on this issue by writing the now classic, *When Bad Things Happen to Good People*. After the birth of his son, Aaron, who was born with progeria (a rapid aging disorder that results in old age death for children in their early teen years), Kushner found himself on the horns of a dilemma. As he tried to understand why this bad thing had happened to his family, his first thoughts were that he had done some "wrong" and God was punishing him. Yet, in review of his life and actions he could find no reasons. The next logical conclusion, was that God was bad and uncaring. Of course, he couldn't accept this perspective. So, why did it happen? Where did he go wrong?

It is indeed, prophetic that after much prayer and reflection, Rabbi Kushner rectified his anguish with a simple, yet power conclusion. This reality for Aaron did not suggest that he or God was bad. Rather, Kushner concluded exactly what was written into the Americans with Disabilities Act (ADA) some 20 years later – that disability is within the natural course of the human endeavor! Aaron's situation, in the scheme of things, was no different than any other uniqueness known to humanity.

This conclusion has offered relief to hundreds of thousands of people, yet it is still not fully appreciated or understood. Indeed, far too many people see the differences associated with disability as tragic aberrations to be offset from our culture and pitied.

TO WHOM DIFFERENCE OCCURS

Another dimension to the question of difference relates to who is on the receiving end of difference. For example, if a pro football player is injured in the course of a game, the difference that might ensue is seen in a disparate way compared to an injury that might befall someone who is drinking and driving. Both injuries might manifest in the exact same type of difference, yet who the injury happened to becomes a key factor in understanding the way people might be seen and/or treated.

I am the wound and the knife;
I am the blow and the cheek;
I am the limbs and the wheel;
The victim and the
executioner.

This nuance of difference is also found when a person who is well known, or a celebrity, becomes different. In some cases, the public image of the person prior to the difference may change the way the person is treated in a post different lifestyle. In these situations, it is safe to conclude that people with higher profiles, who may be perceived as more valuable in the scheme of things, will tend to weather the stigma of difference. A good example of this phenomena is found with people such as Magic Johnson and the late Arthur Ashe. Both of these well-know athletes have (or had) AIDS, a disease with an incredibly negative stigma attached to it. In spite of the current notions of AIDS, both Johnson and Ashe, because of their previous profiles, have hardly been ostracized.

In my book, *Interdependence*, I examined this notion of value and esteem, and how the economic paradigm sets a tone for how people are treated. The economic paradigm puts a premium on performance, thus the person who can do more, or perform at a higher skill level, is usually valued in our society. Consequently, if the person who experiences difference was previously in a highly valued role, their treatment after the difference will usually be higher than another person with the same condition, but was not previously esteemed. Again, the Johnson and Ashe situations offer an example. Less known people with AIDS face wanton discrimination in most walks of life today. Yet, a celebrity is saved from this treatment.

Another dimension in this question of who experiences difference, can be found when the person in question is a minority. It is well documented that minorities, any of the protected groups, are typically more prone to oppression and devaluation. Thus, when a member of a minority, who already is perceived as different from the power establishment, incurs a substantial change in appearance or skill, that person will be more stigmatized than a valued majority in a parallel situation. That is, the experience of difference, as powerful as any other type of minority situation, can be of double consequence when combined with a pre-existing minority situation.

Tied to this example, of course, are women, racial minorities, elders, children, cultural minorities, religious minorities, people with differing sexual preferences, and the like. Any of the members of these groups tend to be further polarized when a situation that pushes difference happen to them.

Indeed, the review of children and difference poses an interesting juxtaposition. We know that children are often victims of abuse and neglect, as their size and immaturity often make them easy targets. In another curious sense, these same factors have a positive influence when difference might befall a child. When people hear or read about children who have been in an accident or have a disease, they often respond with sympathy or compassion. We hear things like, "they are so young" or "they had so much going for them." The most prominent indicator might be the intensity felt at the funeral of a child or young person. Children, indeed hold a unique place in this discussion of who difference happens to.

To a certain extent, women as well, fall in this "between the seams" spot. Similar to children, women are vulnerable to abuse or neglect that might create a posturing of difference. An example might be homelessness. Women are easy targets to be left by husbands or lovers and in the process can be forced into single parenthood, or homelessness. A penetrating exposé of this reality is found in Jonathan Kozol's book, *Rachel and Her Children* (1987). There is an interesting dichotomy to the things Kozol reports. Although people feel a basic sympathy for women in the position experienced by Rachel, their minority status carries some stigma that somehow they are responsible for the difference they now experience.

For both women and children, the vulnerability to abuse can lead to situations of physical and/or psychological disability. That is, if a child or woman finds themselves a target of abuse, they can suffer the scaring effect of difference. Add this on top of their minority status and the weight can be staggering. Clearly, some people are more susceptible to difference, or more effected when the ravages of difference might occur.

DIFFERENCES IN DIFFERENCE

Moving further in this exploration, we must consider the nature of how some things considered different compare with other types of difference. Although it is difficult to rate or equate differences, clearly in the scheme of things some difference is more dramatic than others.

> In spite of every sage whom Greece can show, unerring wisdom never dwelt below; folly in all of every age we see.
> The only difference lies in the degree.
> N. Boileau-Despreaux

One might better understand this assertion in thinking about disabilities that result from an accident or an illness. If you had to rate the following list of disabling conditions, which one might you choose as most impactful to least impactful? Another task might be to rate these conditions from least compromising, to most compromising.

- Blind
- Quadriplegic
- Scaring
- Deaf
- Brain-Injured
- Facial Disfigurement
- Paraplegic
- Hemiplegic
- Lost Limbs

Knowing that our choices on such matters are relative, there is still trends that can be found in such exercise. Indeed, Yuker (1988) and associates have done many studies on attitudes toward people with disabilities. He found that most people displayed various levels of discomfort when confronted with people of varying types of disabilities. The more overt the physical features, the greater the discomfort.

Recently, my brother in law, Joe, had a virus that rested in his eyes. The result was sensitive, and then blurred vision that totally impaired him. He missed a month of work, could not drive, in fact, could not identify people who would come up to him. In the height of his virus attack, Joe and I talked about comparing his situation to other types of disabilities. He felt that for him, and his type of work (Joe is a printer), nothing could be more compromising than losing your vision.

The point of this discussion, however, is not to rate disabilities as much as it is to realize that some types of difference are more socially polarizing than other types. It not only matters when the difference occurs, and who it occurs to, but what type of difference it is as well. In fact, it is commonly accepted in the disability community that a caste system exists. That is, some disabilities are more accepted in society than others.

Again, with all these discussions, remember that there are two major perspectives of difference. One is found with how the individual (or family) who is experiencing the difference feels. The other is how society (or the community) relates to the difference. Both are powerful and highly influential, but to get beyond difference, changes have to occur on both fronts. The person experiencing difference must come to grips with their situation. This is not to say that they have to like it, or even accept it; but they must come to terms with it. Equally, we must understand how and why society feels as they do, and to inspire a higher order of thinking and feeling about difference. Let's examine both issues:

How The Individual Feels

It is bold to assume how people might feel after a serious difference occurs, but I have done enough study to know that, more often than not, the feelings are not good. Typically, people are not pleased to be different. Over the years, I have assembled a flow of how difference seems to manifest. Using research and ideas from people who have studied loss (Kubler-Ross 1969), I am intrigued by the following dimensions related to difference.

Devastation

This is the onset of the difference. It is the point of impact where the change is introduced and alteration occurs. In most of the negative elements of difference, this stage reeks devastation on the person and their family. Usually, the impact of difference is so severe that it totally changes the pattern and flow of all involved.

Denial

After the impact of devastation, an initial element of denial often occurs. This manifests with the sense that this just can't be happening. A number of people who experienced disabling accidents told me they went through a period when they were sure that the event hadn't happened. They couldn't understand why they were dreaming for so long.

Despair

After the person pushes out of denial, a deep sense of despair can often set in. Many people won't eat or talk. They want to be alone and are totally muted by the impact of difference. People have testified that given the difference, life doesn't seem worth living.

DEPRESSION

After a period of time despair gives way to depression. At this stage, the person begins to confront the difference. Enough time has passed as to begin a sense of orientation to the difference, what it means, and its internal and external effects. Depression is a strange phenomena as it moves in moods and impact. One day may be better than the next and often the different person is not sure what each new day will bring.

DELAY

As depression is often unpredictable and difficult to gauge, an inward period of delay may set in. This notion of delay really describes the pace in which the individual gets prepared to directly deal with the difference. The delay period might be brief or could carry on for years.

Inward Flow of Difference

Devastation → Denial ↘ Despair ↓ Depression

Determination ↖ Delay ↙

Dependence ↙

come to terms & begin decision making

DEPENDENCE OR DETERMINATION

As delay finally gives way to action, a person can be pushed one of two ways- toward a state of resign and then dependence on others for survival – or toward a more bold path of determination. Each of these directions show the individual coping with difference, but from a separate perspective.

The entire inward process might be best understood by the following chart:

HOW SOCIETY RELATES TO DIFFERENCE

As a society that promotes commonality, the typical reaction to difference is caution and concern. As we reviewed earlier, the actions of this caution and concern can range from keeping the different person at arms length to down right hostility. These societal actions can be either overt or covert, and can be formal or informal. That is, people can outwardly show their feelings, or hold their thoughts for more private disclosure.

In a more penetrating way, societal reactions to difference can be framed by laws and become cemented in our culture. In these situations, a collection of people can create a feeling that is so prominent as to anchor a society. Either way, the net result of most societal reactions to difference can promote a sense of injustice. This pushes us to think about justice.

Justice. It seems like such a simple concept – so right – so natural. Yet, this notion of justice is an elusive thing. At times, we feel that we are treated in a just way, and then at other times, we may experience what we perceive as an injustice.

Academically, we know that justice is about rights. Indeed, Doubleday Dictionary (1975) defines *justice* as:

1. Being righteous. 2. Fairness. 3. Being 4. Sound reason. 5. Reward or penalty as deserved. 6. The use of authority to uphold what is right, just or lawful. 7. The administration of law.

All these aspects of the definition of justice make sense. We know that justice is about fairness and sound reason. It implies that rights be upheld and that decency to people shall prevail.

Yet, in a more visceral interpretation, we know that this definition is incredibly subjective. For most of us, justice is a concept that applies differently. When we use terms like rights, fairness, and common sense, the immediate next thought then revolves around the person making the judgement. We all have a different sense of the finer points of what is right and wrong, and although our heritage as Americans suggests some common aspect to these themes, for the most part they are variable.

All of us reading these words can recall a time when we have felt injustice. It might have been a feeling of misinterpretation or exclusion, or times when we were not chosen for a job or promotion and felt we were best qualified, or when we were offended by something we read or heard. Deep or not, all of these, and hundreds (if not thousands) of other times, injustice occurs in or around our lives. Forget formal rules of laws, if we perceive injustice, it is then a reality to us.

This whole issue of injustice is further complicated when one party sees themselves as "just doing their job." All through the civil rights movement in the United States in the 50s and 60s, African-Americans pushed the system and were often beaten back, literally and figuratively, by people who were just doing their jobs.

Even today, there is example after example of these differing perspectives of justice. In fact, recently, I had this same type of experience. I was on my way home from a speaking engagement at Lake Tahoe, Nevada. Arriving early in Reno for my flight, I decided to stop on my way to the airport at a neighboring shopping plaza. I was after a Valentine's Day gift for my wife and daughter. With plenty of time to spare, I was sauntering around the plaza stopping here and there, looking for the perfect gift. Now, to really understand this story, you must know that I was dressed very casually. I had just come from the mountains, hadn't shaved that morning, and was sporting my trusty apple cap (a large droopy hat that conjures up thoughts of Ellis Island at the turn of the century). Needless to say, I had a distinct look. After failing in my quest for a gift, I headed to a nearby restaurant for a bite to eat. Once in the eatery, I decided to call home, and headed for the phone. I had just picked up the receiver when two large men approached me, one on either side. In a breath one said, "Reno police. Would you step outside please."

In this day of "America's Funniest Home Videos" and "Candid Camera," you can imagine my reaction. With a wry smile I said, "Yeah, O.K., where's the camera?" The big guy to my right, with his piercing look, was the first tip-off that, just maybe, the Candid Camera set-up was not there.

As I was ushered outside, my other escort asked if I had any weapons on me. Before I could answer, two Reno squad cars, complete with flashing lights, screeched to where we stood. Four uniform police joined the party, and before I knew it, I was surrounded by six, big cops. Now, this video camera thing again flashed through my mind. This time it was the ominous footage of L.A. police beating Rodney King senseless. After a harrowing 10 minutes, I was finally cleared and allowed to get back to my business. This was only after my car and luggage were searched, I was intimidated and embarrassed.

Now, in light of this story, was an injustice levied? Were these police just doing their job? Indeed, there was a robbery in the area, and I was spotted "loitering" in the plaza. Were my rights infringed by the interrogation I experienced?

So, what do we do about this matter of justice? Do we work in detail to interpret a more refined letter of the law to solidify when and how injustice might occur? Do we attempt, as a society, to clearly define right and wrong? The answer to these questions is *yes*. Indeed, as a society, Americans are obsessed with attempting to clarify, through laws, the boundaries of society. We continue to etch deeper lines to guide us in our execution of justice through laws and basic interpretation of justice.

Perhaps the greatest breakthrough in this effort, at least since the Declaration of Independence, was the Civil Rights Act of 1964. If ever there was a law to interpret the parameters of rights and justice it was this landmark measure. Still, in the years that followed the Civil Rights Act of 1964, injustices occurred. As society became more sensitive to peoples' civil rights, the abuses shifted from overt to subtle. There was, and still is, a deep lingering feeling in America that some people have, or should have more rights than others. Old ways die hard.

All around us today, in spite of the '64 Act and others since, are examples of injustice, exclusion, or just plain hate. The charge of racism, sexism, antisemitism, and handicapism are part of the reality fabric of society. Indeed, in one bizarre week in October 1991, most Americans sat glued to the televised U.S. Senate Judicial Committee hearings on now Supreme Court Justice Clarence Thomas where charges of sexism, racism, and high-tech lynching sailed into the living rooms of our nation.

Added to this debate on justice is another duly complex notion – that of equality. Our passion for justice is clearly rivaled by the quest for equality in America. Yet, this concept, too, needs to be examined. The Doubleday Dictionary (1975) states that *equality* is a derivative of the word *equal*, which means:

> 1. Of the same size, quality, intensity, value, etc. 2. Having the same rank, rights, importance, etc. 3. Fair, impartial, just, equal laws. 4. Having the strength, ability, requirements that are needed. 5. Balanced, level, even.

Just as with justice, the idea of equality is one that is evasive. Are people equal, with the same rank? Do we have a balanced and impartial system or society? In fact, how do we even attempt to measure these things? These too, are not easy questions. Even the most basic reviews show time and again that equality, like justice, is one of those elusive butterflies.

Although the ideal of equality sounds good, so many qualifying elements to this concept make it difficult to discern. Our dream is that we are all equal, yet social stratification pushed by age difference, sex difference, cultural difference, and the like obstruct this notion. Added to this are the economic advantages brought by wealth, status, and position. The net effect is that equality is not much more than a myth. As George Orwell (1945) contended in his haunting book, *Animal Farm,* "Some animals are more equal than others."

This review of justice and equality, though cursory, is not meant to be negative. Justice and equality are critical and need to be studied, examined, and defined. It's just that these concepts are taxing to human understanding. People differ in their perspectives on what they mean and how they should be implemented.

WHEN DIFFERENCE OCCURS

Another important factor in looking at difference relates to when the difference occurs. That is, if we think of difference as life changing, then the era in the persons life when the change occurs is critical. To better understand this notion, we must revisit theory on development. It is commonly understood that there is a scheme associated with development – that people follow general stages in their physical, emotional and psychological growth. Each of these stages presents a distinct posture that, if difference occurs, can be influential to the person's future development of how the person deals with difference.

> Let us not go over the old ground, let us rather prepare for what is to come.
>
> *Cicero*

Most people are aware of Sigmund Freud's (1938) stages of personality development. His pioneering work with the facets of personality, the id, ego, and superego, are both legendary and seminal in the field of psychology.

Even with Freud's work being so well known, probably more vital to seeing the link between difference and onset, is the work of Erik Erikson (1980). Erikson's eight stages expanded beyond Freud's concepts and pushed the notion of development to a lifetime endeavor. That is, although Freud outlined personality development he felt that by early adulthood, around age 21-25, the typical person had reached the major experiences for development. Although he felt people developed in the adult years, this development is not fundamental, but predicated on the experiences of the more important childhood years.

Erikson's perspective is that development is a lifetime event and the stages and focus of adult development are as important in the scheme of things. He writes that the pressures, pace and elements of maturity adults feel can be, and often are critical to personal development.

Given the critical nature of the onset of change, I find it instructive to review and examine Erikson's stages of development. As these stages are now classic in the psychological literature, it is easiest to pull a review of them from an excellent source (Wright, 1982). I use this source because along with a review of the stages, Wright also examines elements of virtue. He writes:

Stage 1:
 The first year of a child's life is that period in which the psychosocial crisis of *trust vs. mistrust is* encountered. The key person to whom the child relates is the mother or maternal person. The social institution which preserves and serves the trust quality, or negatively, mistrust, is that of religion. For Freud, this period was categorized as the oral state, but for Erikson it is broadened to more than the "getting" of orality. *In getting, one also learns how to give.* The virtue Erikson sees emerging in this stage is that of *hope*, as over against despondency.

Stage 2:

In early childhood, usually ages two through three, the crisis of *autonomy vs. shame* and doubt is experienced. Beyond the more singular relationship with mother, both parents now become significant to the child's development. The social institution corresponding to this stage in Erikson's scheme is that of law and order, or the political and legal structures of society which define and protect each person's autonomy in relation to any other's autonomy. In Freud's scheme, this period is generally thought as the *anal* stage. Erikson again expands upon Freud's sexual categories to include the holding on to and letting go of many things, such as toys and hair in addition to the bowel movement. The virtue which this stage fosters is that *of will* or willpower vs. impotence.

Stage 3:

In the play stage, generally ages two through four, the psychosocial crisis of *initiative vs. guilt* is lived through. The persons of significance to the growing child expand now to the basic family. The institution relating to this stage is that of economic order, where initiative is offered its opportunity for expression. Again, comparing Erikson to Freud, the latter considered this general period as the *genital* stage. Erikson broadens his consideration to all those experiences of making like and of playing like. Therefore, the emerging virtue of the third stage is purpose which is found in play, purpose as over against passivity.

Stage 4:

During the school years, prior to adolescence, generally thought of as ages five through twelve, the crisis *of industry vs. inferiority* is faced. Those of significance to the developing person now are all persons with whom relationships are established, those of the neighborhood and school environment. The institution of significance to the fourth stage is that of technology, the realm in which industry is encouraged and rewarded. Freud could only call this period between infantile sexual activity and adolescent *puberty the latency period.* For Erikson, it is a time of actually engaging in the process of making things, as school age children are known to do, along with others. The virtue fostered by this developing state is *competence,* as over against the inability to make things.

Stage 5:

Most crucial to the developing person is the adolescent stage of *identity vs. identity confusion.* This is the period in which the significance of peer groups becomes equal to and often greater than the family. The institution of society which corresponds to this developmental stage is that of ideology. For Freud, puberty is the sexual orientation of adolescence. Beyond Freud, Erikson sees the emergence of identity and the sharing of oneself as the mode of being in the world. The emerging virtue is *fidelity* vs. the vice of apathy.

Stage 6:

In young adulthood the crisis faced is that of *intimacy vs. isolation.* Relationships which become significant in this stage usually involve those of the opposite sex with whom love relations develop, but are not limited to marriage partners. Friends, as well as those involved in cooperative and competitive pursuits, are to be included in the intimacy radius of relations. The broad institution Erikson suggests for this stage is simply that of relationships. Geniality was the word used by Freud to describe the post adolescent period, but for Erikson, the mode is broader than just the physical. Intimacy means giving oneself to another while at the same time finding oneself in a new dimension in the process of shared intimacy. *Love* is the emerging virtue, a strength contrasting with withdrawal and isolation.

Stage 7:

In adulthood, one either becomes *generative or absorbed with oneself.* Thus, the crisis of this period is that of generativity. Those persons of significance to adults are the ones with whom labor is shared and divided. Education is the social institution by which adults provide for the development of future generations. *Care is* the virtue which develops with generativity.

Stage 8:

Finally, in old age, the crisis of *integrity vs. despair* is encountered. Erikson sometimes adds the word disgust to despair and the picture becomes clear when one reflects upon those old persons in whom there is either a predominance of integrity or despair and disgust. The whole world is not significant to the developing older person, all of humanity. The social institution which fosters integrity is that of philosophy, or wisdom. One's basic posture towards the world is simply that of *"being."* Having developed through the eight stages, or having been, one can now simply be and face the prospect of not being. That is integrity. The virtue of this stage is that of *wisdom vs. futility.* (pp. 53-54).

Given the nature of this review, we can pause to think about this issue of onset of difference. Clearly, difference has an incredible impact on not only how the different person feels, but on how the world feels about and treats the person as well. Thus, with difference, it matters much if the change occurs to a youngster, adult or elder. How a person experiences a critical difference, and then how the world treats this same person must be acknowledged.

So clearly, who difference happens to can set a powerful stage for the impact and fallout of the difference. Some people, just by virtue of the luck of the draw, will fair better in difference situations, than others. Obviously these realities are deeply rooted, but just our understanding and acknowledgment of them is a stepping stone to getting beyond difference as a society.

If we follow the Erikson stages a number of factors become important. First, the vulnerability to the core development issue as well as the virtue of that same stage must be acknowledged. That is, if difference occurs when a person is going through stage 5, that of identity, the reactions of peer groups to the difference become a critical variable. If the difference, however, occurs at, say, stage 6, the identity issue may be in effect and peer issues may not be as important, but intimacy issues may be affected. Here, the person's vulnerability shifts to the reactions of significant others.

Another factor might be found if the difference occurs before the individual has established a strong pre-difference identity. They will then, more often than not, develop an identity that builds from the difference. In some ways, this might account for the cycle of dependency that sociologists write about when they review generations of families who are dependent on welfare. In these situations, children of poverty develop an identity built from the experience of poverty and then live out the identity.

This type of analysis might also explain why many people with congential disabilities are often passive about the way society treats them, as opposed to people who acquire disabilities later in life. Disability advocates will tell you that the folks who forged a "typical" identity and then experienced a disability through accident, illness or injury tend to be more outspoken and militant about societal devaluation. Clearly onset of difference is an important variable to ponder.

5

Difference and Pity

*Let me set my mournful ditty
to a merry measure
Thou will never come for pity
Thou will come for pleasure*
                        P. B. Shelley

5

Difference and Pity

Another common feature that is often related to difference, revolves around pity. When I write about pity, know that I am referring to the classic features of feeling sorry for someone's situation or plight. The trusty Doubleday Dictionary (1975) defines pity as:

1. A feeling of grief or pain awakened by the misfortunes of others. 2. A cause for compassion and regret.

This definition implies sad feelings caused by someone else's misfortunes. It suggests a key difference between the person with misfortune, and the person who pities. Further, it is a downward emotion with the unfortunate soul at the bottom of the transaction.

To a large extent, when you feel sorry for someone, you pity them. Although this calls forth compassion, an important variable in bridging the gulf caused by difference, it uses compassion in a downward way. When all the cards are cut, no one likes to be pitied – there is something basically devaluing about it.

When I think about pity and difference, I'm called to think about telethons. In this day and age, telethons have become common ways for some charitable organizations to raise money. Although telethons can differ in scope and focus, most telethons use some form of sorrow or pity as a key emotion for soliciting funds. Woven throughout the entertainment or information of the telethon is the basic notion that the persons at the nub of the effort are tragic and the viewing public should give to better their cause.

In his book, *Followers of Jesus*, Jean Vanier (1973) reflects on the spirituality of giving related to pity when he states:

> Compassion is a difficult thing to live... So often, special-ized people are interested in the problem rather than the person, in the handicap rather than the person behind the handicap. These attitudes show a lack of respect and com-passion... They (people who are different) don't want pity, just as they don't want rejection, being looked upon as infe-riors... Giving (through pity) can be a treacherous thing, because by giving we dominate. Those who give must learn also to receive in humility and love and thanksgiving. (pp. 50-51).

To Vanier, people give for a variety of reasons, but when they give from a sense of pity, these gifts can be tainted.

When I see people give out of a sense of pity, it seems that the giver, once the gift has been rendered, is now absolved of any fur-ther responsibility to the person. This notion of absolving is vital to understanding the perversion of pity. If the real goal of an interde-pendent community is to accept and welcome each other, the ab-solving of responsibility is a cancer to the concept. First, it cheap-ens the exchange by putting a dollar sign on responsibility to each other. That is, it lessens the equality between people when one feels obligated to give to another through pity driven by difference. Sec-ond, it drives and reinforces a "we-they" mentality between people. This "we-they" aspect is the direct antithesis of interdependence.

Indeed, researchers in altruism and other types of pro-social behaviors are finding that often, we-they perspective can diminish altruism. In a thoughtful book, titled *The Compassionate Beast*, Morton Hunt (1990) states:

The most obvious fact about altruism is that people tend to practice it toward those in their own group, but not those outside it, for whom they feel anything from indifference to hatred. To some people, their own group can be as large as their society, or even much of humankind; to others it can be as small as their own immediate family. Wherever they draw the line, those within are *we* (the "in group", as social scientists say), one's fellow human beings, who merit help when in need; those outside it are *they* (the "out group"), aliens, who do not. (p. 87)

My concern about telethons or other charitable forms of fund-raising, is that they often draw the line that positions people who have difference as those in the "They" category. The net effect, is that people may give to the charity initially, but by doing so position the recipients of the gift as outsiders.

Another interesting reflection on pity is found in the writings of Ram Dass and Paul Gorman (1985) in their strong book, *How Can I Help?* They write:

Compassion and pity are very different. Whereas compassion reflects the yearning of the heart to merge and take on some of the suffering, pity is a controlled set of thoughts designed to assure separateness. Compassion is the spontaneous response of love; pity, the involuntary reflex of fear. (p. 62)

Dass and Gorman's perspective on pity reinforce this sense of difference and separateness. When we pause to really examine pity we find that it works contrary to interdependence. Still most people continue to embrace pity as a "natural" reaction to difference.

We must work diligently to recognize that difference is difference, nothing more or less. That when we ascribe an emotion, especially a downward emotion such as pity, to difference, the net effect is further polarization and acknowledgment of the factors of difference. We must constantly be attentive to the things that make us similar.

PRE-DIFFERENCE SITUATION

If difference has been thrust upon a person or family, it is important that the pre-difference situation be acknowledged. That is, the lifestyle the person led, how they perceived themselves and how they felt about their situation prior to their difference has powerful impact on the way they will deal with the new experience of difference. This relates to both the internal perspective the person has of themselves, as well as how they think the world views them.

> *Recognize what is before your eyes, and what is hidden will be revealed to you.*
>
> The Gospel of Thomas

Know, in this discussion, I am not referring to the prominent or esteemed person who then encounters difference. We reviewed this in the section on who difference occurs to. Rather, we are looking at the pre-difference situation of the typical person, the average individual who might be hit by a difference.

In my anecdotal experience with difference, this seems true for the people I know. When difference, such as a disability, imposes itself on people, those who had a firm direction in their life seem to have fared better in dealing with the experience. This is not to say that dealing with the difference was easier, only that coping seemed to be more solid.

Further, on the external side, how the now different person was perceived by those around him/her can influence how society might see the person. This factor acknowledges support networks and their importance. Again, for people who had a strong network prior to the difference, the process of dealing with difference seems to follow a stronger profile of adjustment.

If a person led an active lifestyle, full of pace of flow, and then finds themselves confronting a sedentary situation due to the imposition of difference, a number of emotions can follow. It is conceivable that the person could become angry and withdrawn because they now must totally alter their way of life. On the other hand a previously active person may feel that they had good opportunity to participate prior to the experience of difference, and make peace with the change.

An example here, might be a very athletic person experiencing a decline in their skill. As they fade in ability, and see the differences in their competition, some fight the change and try to hang on. Others see it coming and make the best of the change. Neither of these perspectives may be easy, but they do represent the polarities of perspective. Again, in my experience, how people deal with difference, be it insidious or traumatic, has much to do with the person's level of self-esteem and their social support networks prior to or immediately after the change.

To a certain extent, age and maturity must also be factored into this discussion. For the most part, as people age the pace with life changes. A mellowness comes into being and many people find more comfort with the changes that are occurring than a younger person. Again, this is not to suggest that the elder person is happy about shifts and changes in function. Only that there seems to be something about the human condition that softens a perspective on change as one ages.

An interesting lens for this observation is again with my family. As I have shared earlier, I hail from a large Italian family in Pittsburgh. Years ago, my dad and Uncle Sam bought some acreage on a hill that rests above the home that my Grandfather rented. The hill was a humble playground, garden, and private place for the children to learn about life. All the Condeluci children, from my dad to my own children, had their most basic experiences on the hill. With a handshake deal, Uncle Sam and dad bought the hill in 1941 and turned it into a family compound. Today, 15 Condeluci families reside on our hill. Every night, the family elders (my Mom,

Dad, Uncles and Aunts) gather for coffee and pastries at a simple building we call La Cabana. For us, it is paradise, and the Cabana, thanks to Aunt Nat and Aunt Betty, the Condeluci matriarchs, serves as a museum, photo gallery, and place to celebrate meals, events, and happenings.

This is a long-winded way to make a point about the mellowness of aging. Every time we gather, it amazes me how reflective and at peace our family elders are. Know that I have observed these folks for some 46 years. As a large extended family, they have all served, at one time or another, as a parent to me, my brother, sisters and cousins. I remember their vibrancy and powerfulness at family gatherings and events of my youth. Now, as I sit with them, still at times feeling like a child, I marvel at their balance.

My dad is a great example. One of his key goals in life was to have his children settle around him, though he never made any demands. He worked hard to make a living for his family, often holding two or three simultaneous jobs. I know he put a number of his personal dreams on hold for us, most that he was then never able to realize. Today, as his primary goal has been realized, even at the expense of his more personal dreams, he exudes a sense of pride and happiness. Now, I know Dad would be proud if we would have moved off the hill and gone in different directions, still he swells with a sense of accomplishment when he talks about "his" family. We surround him and he often says "now I am at peace, my family is safe and sound."

And so, the Condeluci elders sit in La Cabana for hours and reflect and assess and laugh and cry. It is an incredible, yet simple family ready for the next difference that will arise. Their mellowness serves as a ballast to deal with the inevitable differences and changes that will occur.

All of this, however, underscores the importance of the experiences and stability of the person prior to difference that might occur. People who have a stable, balanced set of experience tend to do better with difference.

Now, this notion of balance and stability is one of real interest to me. How do people become balanced? How do we arrive at a happy point in our lives? I was sitting recently with my friend, Rich Hubert, a fellow I have worked beside for some 21 years now, and we were reviewing the cascade of people we have shared work time with. We both agree to feeling comfortable with over 20 years of tenure with our agency, yet many people we know are still searching. They run from job to job or experience to experience still seeking the next item that will make them happy. Perhaps more money, or a more impressive job title, or more responsibility. These and other items serve to be variables associated with stability and, ultimately, happiness. Yet, are they really?

If balance and stability seem to be variables that help us get beyond difference, we must think them through. What are the items that allow you to feel stable and balance?

RELATING TO DIFFERENCE

So there it is – a basic review and dissection of this notion of difference. It is complex and simple at the same time. It can cause great pain, and lead to incredible perceptions. It can distance us, and yet be liberating. But perhaps the single most prominent feature of difference, is that we all can relate to it. There isn't a person reading these words that hasn't, at some point in time, felt the effects of being different.

> *How can one understand so many things, and put them into practice so little.*
>
> J. Vanier

In an odd way, although difference can offset us from others, it is the great equalizer in that we have all felt it's wrath. From what seems to be simple experiences of childhood (although they were not so simple when we were going through them), to more pronounced experiences of adulthood, to perhaps the more catastrophic situations of accidents or illnesses, or aging, we can all relate.

Indeed, I'd like you to pause now and reflect on a recent (or not so recent) experience of difference. Think back to how it happened, and more importantly, how it felt. Get back in touch with the emotions surrounding the experience and then reflect. How did you feel? Were you avoided or treated in negative ways? Did you have heartache, or shed tears over the event?

Although this kind of reflection can be painful, it is important to call these memories forth to keep balanced as we look to embrace diversity. The last thing you may have wanted when you felt different was to be excluded. Yet, this is often, precisely what we do when we encounter someone who is different from us. We don't know what to say, struggling with our inadequacies that we tend to walk away, or avoid, or just plan ignore.

When you pause to think about it, the awkwardness of difference rolls from two sides. One is the personal feelings of inadequacy, ineptness, ugliness, or whatever else we conjure up as we assess who or what we have become since the onset of difference. These self-pictures that we lay out can be incredibly anchoring. We can constantly remind ourselves that we are different and inadequate that the downward spiral can run out of control. Psychologists call this negative self-talk. It is the feel of negative self-images.

The other phenomena is the awkwardness of friends and associates who struggle to deal with the problem or change that has befallen. I know many people who have experienced the stigma of difference and one common thread of their perspective is how often they are abandoned by friends. Quite simply, those that are close prior to difference often drift apart after the difference occurs. The divorce rate after disability is well documented in the literature as one example of this phenomena.

In my work at UCP, when I talk to those who have drifted due to difference, the former friends tell me they just didn't know what to say, or how to relate to the different person. It is as if the difference overrides the previous friendship.

People with cancer talk often about how friends exit from their life after the diagnosis is made. Again, these former friends state that they just don't know what to say to the person with cancer. Clearly the weight and power of difference can be a painful wedge.

So to me, one way we can hedge against both the way we feel when we are different, and the way others relate to us after difference is to remember our own experiences of difference. This ability to remember can be critical in helping us get beyond the stigma of difference.

This exercise of reflection is not necessarily fun, but it can push us to change our ways. It can get us to personalize. Through a mental renewal of these experiences we can stay conscious to the effects of our behavior when we meet a person who has difference. All of us can do better when we come across people who are different. We can reach out more, smile and welcome more, bridge the gulf that separates. I believe this can only happen when we awaken to the reality of difference.

SECTION II
BEYOND DIFFERENCE

6

Traits For Change

*Discovery consists of looking at
the same thing as everyone else
and thinking something different.*
Albert Szent-Gyorgyi

6

Traits For Change

If you have gotten this far in this book, you have probably experienced, or were touched, by significant difference somewhere in your life. And you know that for us to truly get beyond difference, we must reach even further as a collection of people. We must push ourselves, as a community of people, beyond what appears to be the complexity of difference, to the similarity of being, and an interdependence in activity.

Over the years, society has become more and more hardened and segmented. Clearly, some of this hardening can be seen in our current nature of human services. That is, as our society becomes more sophisticated about difference, it has also become more mechanical about the ways to address difference.

This mechanical nature, I believe, is associated with the medical/expert approach to difference. Earlier in this work, we examined the basic reaction to difference. To grow as people, however, suggests that difference must be more deeply analyzed and studied. We must not let ourselves or our systems evolve to the point where we believe that only the experts really understand any of the difference that we see in today's society.

In fact, if this expert approach does take hold, there is a strong and convincing message to the citizens of our communities. It says, "Don't worry about these different people, experts understand them and can fix them." I submit to you, that this is the wrong message.

Fixing or offsetting is not the way we should deal with difference. Rather, what we need is to understand that all people have a right to be a part of the fabric of community just as they are. And, when we embrace difference, we grow to confront our own humanity. The process liberates us all.

Now, this is an important point to ponder. It suggests that personal growth is launched from a base of security, but fueled by a world of diversity. In my own life, my growth is nurtured by the bosom and security of my family, but stimulated when I meet and interact with people who are different. To a certain extent, the further the difference from me, the more I'm stretched to grow. I believe the same happens, in a collective way, with society.

The operative word in understanding this thesis on growth is *interact*. Note that I did not say react or act, but *interact*. This implies a two-way process – one that pushes and pulls. For most of us, it seems our exchange with difference is to *react*. That is, when we see homeless people our *reaction* is to step aside. When we see people with severe disabilities our *reaction* is to feel sorry. When we see elders our *reaction* is think they are better off in nursing homes or high rises.

When we *interact*, however, the process becomes dynamic. We are pushed to confront or defend the biases or stereotypes we hold about the difference. This testing can then focus our understanding. To this extent, the process becomes liberating and growth enhancing.

Think about it. You don't really understand something until you deal with it, tinker or handle it. This *interaction* leads to understanding and that leads to growth.

The notion of diversity and the harmony found in mixing differences is a unique one that appeals more to the spirit and heart, than to the intellect. In fact, to a certain degree, it forces us to push the other side of complexity. What I mean, is that all of us, regardless of situation, are striving for some basic needs. Maslow's (1968) work suggested a hierarchy of needs starting with the foundation of shelter and physical elements to the more higher order of self-actualization. In the middle of Maslow's scale is, "affiliation or belonging." This need to belong is fundamental to humans. By today's standards, this should be a simple, understood conclusion.

Yet, when difference occurs, we strongly march to the offsetting tune of specialization, creating a framework and wall around the different person that can lead to an exclusion, the opposite of belonging or affiliation. Now, the reasons we do this are complex and a number of them have been explored in this book. In many cases, this complexity becomes so dominant that we get stopped at this point. We keep different people at bay, and create a dualistic approach for goods and services.

This book, however, is about getting beyond this complexity to recognize the simplicity when there is a mixing of diverse variables. Just as with a piano, a single note is simplistic, a cord becomes somewhat complex, but when we apply cords to a complex sonata, they become an active vehicle to an enriched piece of music.

BEYOND DIFFERENCE – TRAITS FOR CHANGE

Getting beyond difference is not an easy task, though. There are powerful forces at work, keeping us hung up in this notion of complexity. Oliver Wendell Holmes once said, "I don't give a figs leaf about simplicity this side of complexity, but I would give my life for simplicity on the other side of complexity." Clearly, Holmes, like so many other great thinkers, knew that achieving simplicity is not an easy thing. He realized that the simple notion of justice is often lost in the complexity of the law. Gandhi, King, and others have written about and reflected on this theme, as well. Most of us can't even understand the question.

So where do we start? How do we come to identify the key elements that are the spring board to getting us beyond difference? As I looked around and talked to many different people, I began to identify a number of important variables. One book, shared values

for a troubled world, (Kidder, 1994) offered eight interesting notions. These are:

Love	Unity
Truthfulness	Tolerance
Fairness	Responsibility
Freedom	Respect

Other authors (Bennett, 1994a; Covey, 1989) explore some of
these and a variety of other virtues and values essential to a strong
character. All of these are important works and worth looking at.
For me, however, I have woven the following Five variables as seminal to getting beyond difference. These are:

Kindness	Hospitality
Generosity	Compassion
Forgiveness	

To this end, consider some spiritual traits that can help us get
beyond difference. They are simple and easy to relate to. In fact, for
most of us they are things we do or have done, but have not applied
to all situations. Know as you look these over, that I am not trying
to preach or convert. It's just that as I have wrestled with attempting to get beyond difference, I have tried the intellectual route only
to be disappointed by what I found. The more I searched for a
clinical formula to help people become included, the more I seemed
to be polarized by the very process. This failure and frustration has
now led me down a different path. It's almost as if I have been
reunited with the most basic of elements and in these, I now see
hope for an answer.

Recognize too, that although these traits all have a spiritual fla-
vor to them, I use the term spiritual with a little "s." In fact, a good
way to couch this entire section is under the heading "secular spiritualism." It's not about converting people or proselytizing. Indeed,
this discussion is purely secular. We each need to consider theology

in our own way. I am convinced, however, that all these traits have a spiritual link in that they all deal with the stuff of relationships and how we position ourselves in this universe. They are about inclusion.

Over the years, I have become increasingly interested in spirituality – what it means, how it affects us as people. As my awareness has grown, I have become amazed at how often I find references to spirituality in readings and literature. Einstein (1956), in his more reflective writings has firmly acknowledged spirituality as key. He stated, "All of science is but a blunt instrument if it does not have behind it a living spirit."

Carl Sagan and Ann Druyan (1992), both well known scientists state:

> If the universe really were made for us, if there really is a benevolent, omnipotent, and omniscient God, then science has done something cruel and heartless, whose chief virtue would perhaps be a testing of our ancient faiths. (p. 413)

Indeed, many of the esteemed scientist, past and present, acknowledge the spiritual side of the ledger. A recent review of self-esteem, conducted in California, suggested that spirituality refers to experiencing ourselves in relationship to the universe." (CTFR,1990). This, to me, is a good baseline to the word and concept.

So join me now as we turn attention to some key traits that combat the negative residue that surrounds difference. If more of the elements of these traits were in play today, we could, as a society, get beyond difference!

7

*K*indness

We are supported to preach
without preaching not by words,
but by our example, by our
actions. All works of love are
works of peace.

Mother Teresa

7

*K*indness

As we explore the five springboard spiritual traits to get beyond difference, all of them, kindness, hospitality, generosity, compassion and forgiveness, are related and work together. Each, as well, stand alone. As I have been reflecting and exploring all five, I have often asked myself, which is the most basic, the one that supersedes or precedes the others?

Now, this is a crazy reflection, probably one that is pushed more by my nature to order things, than by common sense. It seems we always try to find the first, or to proclaim the start point. I know that all five are equally important and related. Still, if I had to select the one that I think should be first, sort of in a friendly way, it would be kindness. When I think of basic, folksy, spiritual notions, I think of kindness.

I'm not sure why this is, but I know that I reflect on it a lot, and I know that I try to be more tuned into kindness in my own life. Kindness – it's one of those concepts that is both simple, yet elegant.

Certainly, kindness is a close cousin of hospitality. One of my friends suggests that hospitality is the child of kindness. When people are kind, it is easier to be hospitable. They suggest that kindness is a core and hospitality is the action.

I'm not sure of this, but I know that I find myself talking more about kindness with my children than any of the other four traits, even though they are all important. Again, not that there is some competition, but that it is just easier. It is a simple concept, to be kind, and my children can understand. When I suggest that they be compassionate, or hospitable, or generous, they struggle more to understand. But with kindness, they know what I mean and can relate.

The first issue with kindness rests with a definition. What does it actually mean? When I pose this question to friends or students, they first seem taken aback. Everyone knows what kindness means- to be nice, gentle, agreeable. So what do you think, what is kindness to you?

Perhaps, to help in this exercise, try thinking of the kindest person you know. What is it about this person that makes them kind? How do they carry themselves? What colors their actions? Can we only tell if people are kind through their actions? Are there some people you meet who you just know are kind, even before they demonstrate kindness?

So, what is kindness? How is it formally defined? The American Heritage Dictionary (1992) says:

> *Kind-ness.* 1. An act or instance of being kind. A favor. 2a. The quality or state of being kind. 2b. A feeling of fondness. *Kindness.* 1. The state or quality of being kind. 2. A kind act; favor. 3. Kind behavior. 4. Friendly feeling; liking.

These definitions help us understand that kindness is an active phenomena. In fact, all five traits examined in this work, require an action on the part of the person. To be kind implies that there is an act. The definition also implies that acts alone are not tantamount to kindness. Rather, kindness happens when the person reaches a level of quality or, as they say, a state of being kind.

Along with this definition of kindness, comes the elements that surround kind acts. That is, are there calculated precepts to a kind act? Do people act the way they do because they have a hidden agenda?

When I think of this question, I am drawn to recall an experience I had in Philadelphia a few years back. I had to make a presentation in the city of Brotherly Love and arrived at the airport late on a rainy Saturday night. Since I don't like to take cabs when I travel, I stopped a sky cap to ask about public transit options. He told me I could get to the city by bus, but I must make a tricky connection to the subway at Veterans Stadium. I was struggling to understand the directions when a strange-looking man stepped from the shadows and announced that he was going downtown by bus and would escort me. Just as I was sizing him up, piercing eyes, need for a shave and rumpled clothes, a bus pulled up and he said, "This is our bus."

He got on and turned to look at me from the steps. Bags in hand, I must have had a foolish look on my face as I followed him onto the empty bus. Could I trust this man? Would he be kind? Was I taking too great a chance?

As the bus moaned away from the terminal we sat down. He looked me over and asked what type of work I do? I mumbled some transparent answer and really began to feel that I had made a serious mistake. With the rain and fog outside, he, I, and the bus driver inside, I'm sure we created a surrealistic image that only Fellini could have appreciated.

Soon, we came to a stop and he announced that this was our point of departure. We both stood up and descended into a rainy dark bus stop. As the bus departed, he guided me to an area that led to the subway steps. I could see a foggy image of Veterans Stadium and I remember commenting on some inane sports issue as we descended the steps.

Quietly, we made our way through a dark subway station. Soon, a train came and he guided me in. By this time, I could read the headlines in tomorrow's Philadelphia Inquirer, "Pittsburgh Man Found Slain in Empty Subway Station." In the train, he asked me what hotel I was at and I couldn't believe myself when I answered. He said he was going further, but would see me to my hotel. Before I could protest that I didn't want to put him out, the train stopped and he guided me out.

As we arrived at street level, he pointed to my hotel just across the way. Then he asked me if I would be taking the subway/bus back to the airport when my conference was concluded. With a curious look on my face I answered, "yes." As he dug his hand into his pocket, I was sure the anticipated challenge, a knife or gun, was now to occur. You could imagine my surprise when he pulled from his pocket and handed me a subway token. He told me to take it, it would expedite my trip back.

As I took the token I asked him how much I owed him. He looked at me with those piercing eyes and paused an eternity. Then he said. "Just do something kind for someone, sometime," and then disappeared into the night.

Walking into the lobby of the hotel, I had a strange feeling. It had to be the same sense that Carlos Castaneda had when he met Don Juan. You just never know when those acts of kindness are going to occur, and how your life may be effected by the act.

When I told a friend about this story, she paused and then reflected on how it took my generosity of acceptance to bring out this persons gesture of kindness. Now I not sure if my actions were generous or stupid. In an innocent way, I hoped that this stranger would be honest and helpful in the transaction. To my friends point, I'm not sure kindness is dependent on generosity, but it does take an active recipient on the receiving end of a kind act.

I still think about the experience in Philadelphia and the strange man on the bus. In fact, he pops into my mind at times when I am not as kind as I might have been. He looms as a messenger of kindness for me and, at times, reminds me to "do something kind for others." What an experience and what a gift.

A friend in Kansas, when I recalled this story, asked me if I used the token to head back to the airport. I admitted I had and he thought I would have been wiser to have saved it as a symbol of kindness. Although this is a warm thought, one I wish I had followed up on, just my recollection of this event, the opportunity to tell others about it, is surely a second best use of my Philadelphia friend's kindness.

Another interesting aspect of kindness, revolves around wholeness. That is, can people be selectively kind? Can you show kindness to one group or on one issue, but not on another. Some people I talked to on this topic said yes, others argued no. My daughter, Gianna, told me, you're either kind, or your not, you can't ride the fence on kindness.

It has always amazed me when people demonstrate kindness to people that they know or love and then turn an angry tone to others. I remember watching the PBS series, *Eyes on The Prize* with my children a few years ago. This documentary chronicled the civil rights movement with amazing footage of atrocities for those who challenged the Jim Crow laws of the South. Scene after scene showed angry white mobs shouting obscenities at school children in Little Rock, or bus riders in Jackson, Mississippi or peaceful marches in Selma, Alabama. My children asked, "Daddy why are those people so mean?" I tried a feeble answer, but what shocked me was that these same people, the ones shouting obscenities, would then tuck their children into bed lovingly, or attend church on Sunday as if nothing happened. How could people be tender and kind one moment and then have hate flow from them the next?

Similarly in a recent tour of the U.S. Holocaust Museum in Washington, D.C., one cannot get through this exhibit without wondering why the violence and hatred? As I looked at photo after photo of the desecration, I found myself peering into the eyes not of those persecuted, but of the Nazis. How could these people be totally oppressive to the Jews and other non ayrans and then be kind to their family and friends? Even some seemingly logical of explanations of politics, nationalism, economic decline and other factors defy, in my mind, that stark differentiation in kindness and hate.

It's interesting to consider kindness in today's world. In some instances, we are witnessing strong messages of exclusion, hate, and dispassion. In the name of a better world, some people are arguing that certain groups are not welcomed into the agenda. In fact, the resurgence of hate and violence to people who have certain types of difference, is rising today at an alarming rate. As I write these words, neo-nazis in Germany are terrorizing foreigners and religious minorities. These hoodlums, dubbed "skin-heads" are waving swastikas and singing chants in praise of Adolph Hitler.

In another area of the world, Bosnia Herzegovina, an ugly predicament has occurred where Muslims, Serbs, and Bosnian people leash out at each other. Reports in the area talk about "ethnic cleansing" where Serbs have carried out a systematic agenda of torture, rape and murder of Muslims and Bosnians all in an effort to clean out undesirables.

Closer to home, in America, the Pittsburgh Post-Gazette (James, April 11, 1993) reported some alarming figures. The White Aryan Resistance, or WAR estimates that there are some 3,500 neo-Nazi skinheads in Southern California alone. Further, the Ku Klux Klan reports some 6,000 members, many living in the northeast and midwest. Add on to this the 1,000 more hard-line racists associated with the Aryan Nations and the numbers of those who are intolerant become very alarming. In fact, the article in the Post-Gazette suggested there are some 150,000 active hate mongers, spread out in some 346 separate organizations, each with their own structure, by-laws and leadership.

This same article goes on to point out that California alone hosts 30 hate groups, followed next by Florida with 20. Pennsylvania, Illinois, and Georgia are in third place with 18 each, then Michigan 16, Texas, 15, Tennessee, 13, Oregon, 12, then New Jersey, Ohio and North Carolina each with 11. So clearly, no particular region of United States has a monopoly on organized hate.

Another frightening reality, and one that seemingly goes beyond hate, is the phenomena of people who do violent acts against others for no apparent reason. A front page article in the Philadelphia Inquirer (December 6, 1992) reported on what they called "A new generation of killers, ones who feel no blame and no shame." The reporter reviewed 57 cases of teenagers charged with murder. Of the 18 killers that they did an extensive interview with, every one saw themselves as not responsible for the murder. These kids blamed the victims for not following the rules of violence. It is also important to note that most of these killers did not have viable family guidance; they were kids of the streets.

In a Newsweek article, titled "Wild on the Streets" (Kantrowitz, August 2, 1993), some unbelievable statistics and trends on violence are reported. The author states:

> Between 1987 and 1991, the number of teenagers arrested for murder around the country increased by an astounding 85 percent, according to the Department of Justice. In 1991, 10- to 17-year-olds accounted for 17% of *all* violent crime arrests; law enforcement officials believe the figure is even higher today... According to the FBI, more than 2,200 murder victims in 1991 were under 18- an average of more than six young people killed everyday... Each year nearly a million young people, between 12 and 19 are raped, robbed or assaulted, often by their peers." p. 43

This kind of data is sad to report in any context, but in conjunction with a discussion on kindness it seems overwhelming. How can there be such a rise in actions that go against the grain of the very basic lessons that most everyone reading this book had learned at an early age? Why does it seem so easy to hate? How can people, using an indicator such as religion or color of skin, disobey those basic lessons from mother?

No one knows for sure, but clearly we can speculate. To be kind calls on our sense of security. The more a person is secure, the easier it seems to be able to reach out to others. Now, when I raise the issue of security, especially in the context of this section on traits, know that I am referring to spiritual security. Often, we think of security from a material sense, and indeed, some acts of kindness rise from material security. But for the basic act of kindness, material wealth or security is not a necessity. Rather, for kindness to occur the initiator must be spiritually secure. They must be ready to accept that through their act of kindness the recipient might take advantage of them, and if that happens, so be it. It seems that many people just can't take that risk.

And so, kindness requires risking; a willingness to be nice even if there is no direct return for the act. Yet, when we really stop to examine kindness, especially the actions of kindness, amazing things happen. I know for me, when I started my deeper inquiry into all the five traits explored in this book, my consciousness was pricked. I became more attuned to kindness, more aware of its place in our culture.

This consciousness raising is an important exercise. Somehow, we have become so conditioned to the negatives of society, like the statistics reported in Newsweek or the Pittsburgh Post-Gazette, that we lose track of all the kind acts that happen daily. As my sensitivities heighten, I am constantly encouraged by these actions. Some are large and heroic, others small and less dramatic, but all are signs of hope.

Like a couple weeks ago, I was invited to make a presentation about the United Way to a team of campaign chair people at the University of Pittsburgh. Since my organization, UCP, is a recipient of United Way dollars, I am often asked to share ideas and stories with donor groups. Further, the University of Pittsburgh is a major employer in our city there were close to 250 chair people in attendance.

As the guest speaker, a seat was held for me in the front of the room with the University chancellor and other dignitaries. We were sitting for breakfast before the ceremonies and I was across from the chancellor. Our table was full, save one seat. As we were chatting I noticed that the chancellor was looking closely at a table off to the corner. I glanced that way, as well, and noticed that one young person was sitting alone at a large table. When I looked back toward the chancellor he was gone. I thought he might be about working the crowd, perhaps he had seen a Dean, or other dignitary that he needed to acknowledge. Then I saw that he was headed over to the corner table.

In a blink, he was back to our table escorting the person who was sitting alone. He asked her to sit and introduced her around our table. I was sure, In spite of her young age, that she must be an important person and one that the chancellor needed to impress. As it turned out, she was a clerk in one of the departmental offices, hardly a dignitary to be courted. I had thought that, although the chancellor's act was a kind one, it must have had some calculated aspects to it. Instead, he was just reacting with a sense of kindness and hospitality to someone who was alone. It was a literal translation of "do onto others as you would have them do unto you."

Kindness is always sweeter when it is least expected. Someone who offers a hand when it is most needed, or a soft word when you're down or a smile when your day is sour. Time and time again, I am encouraged by acts of kindness to me or those that I observe around others.

I have a friend who contends that kindness differs from generosity because generosity mandates that something tangible, money, gifts, time, etc. must pass hands. Kindness, on the other hand, doesn't require tangible things, but can be more intangible in nature. Like with the University chancellor example, it cost him nothing to invite the person to our table. If it had, my friend would contend that it wasn't an act of kindness, but of generosity.

Now, I am not sure if this tangible/intangible issue is a line of demarcation between kindness and generosity. It does seem that kindness might be a precursor to generosity. That is, does one have to be kind in order to be generous? In the same vein, can one be kind without having to be generous? Or, can one be generous without being kind?

Yet, kindness does require action. In fact, how can we really know if a person is kind until they act. Even an action as simple as a smile requires that something actually occurs. Without an action phase, kindness is just a hollow word.

Another dimension might revolve around the notion of a kind act. Just what is a kind act? If someone smiles at you, does that constitute a kind act? Someone once told me that occasionally, when he is driving on a toll road, he will pay the attendant for his car and the one behind him, even though he doesn't know the person. He says doing this makes him feel good, just trying to imagine how the person behind him might feel. I don't know; is this a kind act or humorous speculation to the other person's reaction?

Indeed, I recently came across the book, *Random Acts of Kindness* (1993). This book examines acts of kindness levied toward those you do not know. It suggests that the more we can do this, the better off our society will be. I know that this type of book is found in the popular literature base, but we'd all do better to study it's contents diligently.

Others I talk to, tell me that kindness is often distinguishable through actions. That when people do things for others, especially when there is no direct pay out for them, this can be one hallmark of kindness. Take, for example, my mother-in-law, Concetta. For a number of years, she would bring soup weekly to a neighbor who became shut-in. In this situation, "Coungy," as she is affectionately known, had nothing to gain as her neighbor was poor, with no family network. Now I know, from over 30 years of observing Coungy, that she is indeed, a kind person. She constantly extends to others and is incredibly selfless. Recently, I asked Coungy about her actions, why she brought the soup. She seemed amazed that I would ask such a question and after a short pause she said, "It's the least I could do for her."

My sister-in-law, Marie suggested an interesting perspective to me, when she offered that kindness is influenced by mood. Although Marie is a kind person, she tells me that it is easier for her to be kind when she is in a good mood. Are people who are kind because they are in a good mood, really kind people? That is, if you're only kind when you are in a good mood, is this truly kindness?

On the other side of this same issue, does being kind keep people in good moods? I don't know how empirical this is, but it seems to me that kind people are often in good moods. In fact, as I sit here and type these words, I am trying to think of one kind person I know, who is not usually in a good mood. I can't think of a one.

Maybe this is a good test to try yourself. Do some kind things for people around you and keep track of your moods. Although this would be an interesting study, I'm sure most human service researchers would scoff at the idea.

My wife, Liz, recently told me a story of kindness that she witnessed. She was on an excursion to the mall and while in the store she saw two people speaking loudly and harshly to a person who appeared to have a disability. Knowing about organized human services, Liz thought the two folks must be staff of some group home and the person at the brunt of their tirade was a client. She watched for a while and these two "staff" were still being rough, seemingly beyond need. Before Liz could intervene another woman approached them and asked what was going on. Sure enough, the two people identified themselves as staff of a nearby group home. Still, the women persisted, she wanted them to show some identification and why they were being so rough. They reluctantly gave information to the woman, but before she would stop her inquiry she wanted to call their agency, just to make sure.

Now here was a total stranger, with no vested interest except the well being of a vulnerable person. Why did this person step forward, what was her motive? What could she gain from this interchange? Was it that she was just in a good mood?

It seems to me, as we dig deeper into kindness, some very basic elements emerge. Although the issues of motive, payoff, or even mood, might have some influence on kindness, they are not seminal factors of kindness. There seems to be some more basic elements of kindness that some people have more of than others.

When I presented this idea to a friend of mine, he said, "So what! Why make such a big deal out of it? Who cares why people are kind? We should be more concerned if they aren't. If some people are kind because of a motive, at least they are kind at all."

My friend's simplistic analysis of all this does shift me to another thought about kindness. That is, can we develop kindness in ourselves? Indeed, can a person who is not prone to be kind, become kind in a conscious endeavor? My cleric friends tell me yes. That in some regards, this is one objective of organized religion.

Now it seems that if kindness is vital to helping us get beyond difference, and getting beyond difference is a route to interdependence, then the kindness enhancement business must happen over and above organized religion. By this I mean, that we should look for more opportunities to have our "kindness consciousness" raised. We can't leave this all to the churches. One reason is that not all people go to church, or if they do, some don't really hear the message. Another reason is that even for those who do go to church, and pay attention, other things creep into our consciousness and we quickly forget.

One way to come to know kindness better, is to talk about it, ferret out its innuendos. I did this recently with a class I teach for Allegheny County Community College. I asked my students to define kindness in a word and here is what they said:

Kindness is:

caring	cheerfulness
gentleness	respect
fairness	helping others build
sensitivity	loving
giving	acceptance
happiness	listening
always there	constructiveness

One of the students thought that people must first be kind to themselves before they can be kind to others. The student felt that without the basic level of security, kindness could not really happen. Another student argued however, that he knows a number of people who had very ugly experiences, and this history caused them to be hard on themselves, unkind in a way, yet terribly kind to others. He felt this type of overcompensation was still bonafide acts of kindness.

Although these seem to be simple conclusions, they are important elements for reflection. In our Beyond Difference class, we took the time to analyze and reflect on these simple notions. As we did, it became apparent that these simple themes were indeed complex. But isn't that always the case, where basic items are the most difficult to understand?

Often, with kindness, I am reminded of the golden rule — do unto others as you would have them do unto you. Such simple advice, and profound as well, yet so difficult to truly live. A person I met at a recent presentation, put a nice twist on the golden rule. He said he added a clause to the rule and tries to live by it. He told me, "Do unto others as you would have them do unto you, but do it first!" What a neat idea – to make the golden rule proactive!

I had a recent golden rule experience at home that was unique. A few weeks ago, I overheard my two boys, Dante and Santino, playing in the back room. As often happens, their play started to accelerate and before too long their voices raised and then out of the back room ran Santino, crying. He told me Dante had pushed him down. I called Dante in to investigate the allegation. Being five years older than Santino, he often overpowers him. I asked Dante to explain what had happened. He said, "Dad, I was only doing what I heard you talk about all the time." I said, "Oh, what is that?" He paused a few minutes and said, "Do unto others as they do unto you – Santino pushed me, so I pushed him back!" I could hardly hold back the laughter as I clarified the golden rule. Funny, though, the more I look around the more I seem to see people using Dante's interpretation. As old as the golden rule is, we still struggle to understand it.

Clearly, there is much more to the discussion of kindness. It is a simple concept, but has a complex interior. As we move through the rest of these springboard traits to get beyond difference, know that the agenda is not to tell readers how to be kind, but rather to raise general questions of kindness in hope that we can find our own way.

8

Hospitality

8

Hospitality

What a warm, welcoming concept the word hospitality conjures up. We hear of it in national ads for large hotels, see it in family gatherings, tell our children to be hospitable, yet how often do we pause to understand, or more importantly, practice this concept.

Before looking more closely at hospitality, lets define it. Here's a couple definitions that I found.

> *Doubleday Dictionary* (1975) – Welcoming and entertaining guests with generous kindness; open minded and receptive.
>
> *Webster's Third New International Dictionary* – 1a. the cordial and generous reception and entertainment of guests or strangers socially or commercially 1b. an instance of hospitality 2. Ready receptivity especially to new ideas and interests.
>
> *American Heritage Dictionary* (1992) – 1. The friendly reception and treatment of guests or strangers; an act or show of welcome. 2) The quality of being hospitable and welcoming to guests or strangers.

These definitions revolve around some interesting and basic themes. They speak to welcoming people, friendships, openness to guests, receptivity to new ideas, generosity, and cordiality. In a way, they inspire a notion of warmth and format where there are no strangers. They cause us to think through our relationships with others and offer a fine primer for an abstract understanding of hospitality. Yet, most of us really learn about hospitality first at home, our initial teachers being our parents and family. This type of learning is through observation and constancy. We come to know a concept by watching those that we trust and love play out the theme.

Of course, the romantic notion of how we learn hospitality can also be found in the old neighborhood examples we see in the movies or read in books. You know the ones, where each person in the neighborhood knew each other, and sat outside on porches to listen to the ball games on the radio, watched out for each other. Baked goods were exchanged and people were truly connected.

But how many people today can remember or can relate to this method of learning hospitality? The suburban community where people may not even know their neighbor seems to be the reality today. To this point, I was recently in California to do a presentation. Late one day, I went outside to the pool, hoping to take advantage of the nice weather. Trying to keep up with my writing, I had my trusty laptop handy, hoping to pound out some new ideas (I thought the sun would inspire me). Not long after I sat down, another guest of the hotel, in true quest of the sun, took a lounge chair near me. Soon we were talking. I was fumbling with this notion of community, neighborhoods, and hospitality, and told him about my ideas. I talked about Condeluci Hill and my neighborhood. I told him that I thought community and hospitality were things that people needed.

He was amazed that I would think that people can, or even should, spend time with their neighbors. Then he told me that he had been living in his Los Angeles community for the past three years and did not even KNOW his neighbors. Can you imagine that? Three years and he had no clue of who was around him – on both sides.

Now, I don't know about you, but I can't understand this. I appreciate that he lives in Los Angeles, and I know that things are different there. But come on, three years and no connections. I asked him, and I know it was none of my business, but I had to know; who did he connect with? He told me he had many friends and was into many associations, but in Los Angeles, these were linked by freeway. Indeed, he had community in his life, not geographic, but more topical in nature. His community revolved around his interests and his "neighbors" were people with similar interests.

Now, stop for a moment to think how people in this type of experience might come to practice hospitality. Doors in communities locked up tight, neighbors off on the freeway to connect in some offset place. It is as if one wants to practice hospitality they need to consciously travel to the settings where friends might gather. This is clearly not "stuff" of the romantic settings of Brooklyn, South Philadelphia, or Brookline in Boston, where people are more closely linked, and have opportunity to practice hospitality over their backyard fence.

As I talked to my new friend about the differences in these notions of community, it caused me to think further to focus the role of hospitality. It became clear that this notion of traditional community needs to be better understood. In his thoughtful monograph, *Building Community*, John Gardner (1991), identifies the concept of traditional community. He states:

Setting about the contemporary task of building community, one discovers at once that the old, beloved traditional model will not serve our present purposes well. Nostalgia for "the good old days" will not help us through the turbulent times ahead.

The traditional community was homogeneous. Today, most of us live heterogeneity, and it will inevitably affect the design of our communities. Some of the homogeneity of traditional communities was based on exclusionary practices we cannot accept today.

The traditional community experienced relatively little change from one year to the next. The vital contemporary community will not only survive change but, when necessary, seek it.

The traditional community commonly demanded a high degree of deformity. Because of the nature of our world, the best of our contemporary communities today are pluralistic and adaptive, fostering individual freedom and responsibility within a framework of group obligation.

The traditional community was often unwelcoming to strangers, and all too ready to reduce its communication with the external world. Hard realities require that present-day communities be in continuous and effective touch with the outside world, and our values require that they be inclusive.

The traditional community could boast generations of history and continuity. Only a few communities today can hope to enjoy any such heritage. The rest, if they are vital, continuously rebuild their shared culture and consciously foster the norms and values that will ensure their continued integrity.

In short, much as we may value the memory of the traditional community, we shall find ourselves building anew, seeking to reincarnate some of the cherished values in forms appropriate to contemporary social organization. The traditional community, whatever its shortcomings, did create, through the family, through the extended family and through all the interlocking networks of community life a structure of social interdependency in which individuals gave and received support — all giving, all receiving. With that no longer available, we must seek to reconstruct comparable structures of dependable interdependency wherever we can — in the workplace, the church, the school, the youth-serving organizations, and so on. (pp. 11-12).

Like it or not, the primary lessons of hospitality are innocently rooted in the day-in day-out practices with those closest to us and usually these are our families and the neighbors in our lives. Gardner admits that the basics of community are changing, but the interdependency of people will always remain. Through these interdependencies, we will find hospitality.

I don't reflect on this to be critical or to run down a more distanced, suburban lifestyle; only to comment on the changing face of how we become acquainted with, and then understand hospitality. I am sure there are some advantages for children growing up in settings like the one experienced by my friend in Los Angeles, but it seems so fast paced; out of sync. For me, as I imagine for most of you, the starting point of understanding this notion of hospitality is found in our family, and to a large extent, our neighborhood and community experiences. This enculturation of hospitality creates a basic understanding, and for the most part, happens so insidiously, that we are hardly aware of the experience. When did we first learn hospitality? Indeed, how did we learn to be hospitable? More basically, what is hospitality?

In my quest to better understand hospitality, I have raised it in question with people I come in contact with. Recently, in a workshop I conducted on this concept of difference, I posed the question of hospitality to my class. After an initial discussion, I again asked the participants to define hospitality in a word. Here's what they told me:

Hospitality means:

open	welcoming	excited
unselfish	at home	belonging
loving	accepting	shelter
warmth	not on a schedule	inviting
generous	comforting	unconditional

I asked these same students to call forth the person in their lives that most embodied hospitality. I wanted them to see that person in their minds and to hear their voice. Then I asked them about this person. Out of class of 25, 60% of the students saw a woman, about 50% saw a relative or spouse and about 30% saw a younger person (under 30). Who would you see in such an exercise? Most importantly, what is it about this person that makes them stand out?

ACTIONS OF HOSPITALITY

As I think about hospitality and ways to operationalize this spiritual concept, a number of themes come to mind. These are:

Touching	Being upbeat
Nurturing	Extending to others
Being attentive	

Of course, there are others, but for me, these items stand out. Here are some things I've come to know on these issues:

TOUCHING

Given the uniqueness of my culture and life on "Condeluci Hill," I had a number of aunts and uncles, all who served, at one point or another, as teachers and guides. What a beautiful opportunity this afforded my brother, sisters, cousins, and I to the features of hospitality. First, to observe how my relatives handled each other, and then how they related to strangers. In all regards, my first thoughts of hospitality revolve around touching. There was always touching, hugging, and kisses. Even with strangers, I remember the warm, two-handed handshakes or arms draped around the shoulder. There was never a doubt that my parents, uncles and aunts were truly happy to meet a new person. In cases where the stranger is a friend of one of my family, the person is treated almost the same as that family member would be treated.

This notion of touching and hospitality is striking. It is always intriguing for me when I meet new people or observe two people meeting for the first time. In fact, I am a student of observing these interchanges. As I do my observation, an important point to know, or to guess, is who the host may be. In most new connections, usually one person plays the role of host, and the other as guest. How the host reaches to greet, and make contact with the guest is the first major exchange of hospitality.

As I observe, or participate, some people are clearly more fluid, and physical than others in greeting and touching. Why is this? Clearly, not all people have stopped to study, or practice hospitality. Most people just go to automatic pilot in these experiences. So what is it that allows one person to physically greet and touch a stranger, making them feel really welcomed; when another person may seem to be inept, or uncomfortable in this type of exchange?

Now it's important to note that touching does drift into some personal dimensions. Some people are comfortable touching – others are clearly uncomfortable. As a "toucher" myself, I am always amazed and sometimes amused at people's reaction to my touching. Some are open and welcoming and others put signals and space that announces they do not want to be touched.

Over the years, scientists and researchers have examined aspects of touching (Montagu, & Matson, 1983; Morris, 1971), and they differentiate between social and intimate touching. There are barriers and borders that play out when examining the phenomena of touching. Still, with hospitality, the handshake, hug, arm around the shoulder, and pat on the back are all basic signals of hospitality.

A great place to explore touching and hospitality from afar, is at the airport. Since my work takes me around the country, I have had numerous chances to study hospitality in this venue. It is intriguing to find the myriad of expressions at airports. Some people politely shake hands, others warmly embrace, while still others swoop onto each other and spin around. I love this last type of exchange. It shows an unedited expression of hospitality. Now I understand that who we greet is as important as how we greet. Still, most of us follow a basic script.

One important factor related to touching can be tied to cultures and customs. Some cultures are more stoic, further removed than others. This might have nothing to do with personal warmth, only that the culture keeps more space between the players.

A few years ago, I had an experience that drove home this important point of customs that affect touching. I met a warm woman at a conference and she was engaged with the concept of interdependence. We exchanged phone numbers and over the ensuing months had a number of good conversations about barriers toward interdependence that we had at our organizations. We had a good rapport and soon she wanted me to lead a discussion with the staff at the rehabilitation hospital where she worked. When I arrived on the arranged day and saw her in the lobby I moved to give her a hug, a way I typically say hello to people who are "kindred spirits." To my amazement, she jerked back from my advance saying she couldn't give me a hug. In an awkward rebound, I asked if we could shake hands and she said no. I was clearly off balance until she told me her religious convictions allowed her to touch no man but her husband. It was an interesting sensitizing experience for someone who takes hugs for granted.

Think now, about how you move to greet newcomers. What are your actions? Do you show a genuine interest in the new person? How do you show affect? What are the physical features of your hospitality; can you identify them?

NURTURING

Next in hospitality, to me, comes the importance of physical nurturing. Often, after greetings and physical contact, comes an invitation to eat or drink together. My Aunt Nat, one of our family matriarchs (and my Godmother) is an artist in hospitality. Her warmth and sincere interest in people she meets offers a lesson to us all. Immediately after the introductions, Aunt Nat always asks, "What can I get for you?" Be it coffee, or pastries, a full meal or just a warm seat, Aunt Nat knows about hospitality.

In preparing for this book, I asked Aunt Nat to reflect on hospitality, to think back to how she learned to welcome people. She warmly recalled from the early experiences at her mother's feet, the essential nature of tending to others. Any time a newcomer would enter their home, Aunt Nat's mom (my grandmother) would rush to make them feel

> *The first step in the evolution of ethics, is a sense of solidarity with other human beings.*
> A. Schweitzer

at home. Even though her family was poor, there was always coffee, bread, wine, and leftovers that were ready to be heated and served. Along with the nurturance of food, the Condeluci homestead was also rich in spirit, especially in good conversation and music. Story after story followed that tied in the ingredients of food/drink, strong conversations, and the joy of music and dance. Grandpa with his concertina (a type of accordion) and Grandma with her tambourine topped off many a great evening with guests in song.

These reflections of Aunt Nat are consistent with many others who I have talked with. Often, after I do presentations that include a discussion of hospitality, many a person approach me to talk about their experiences. The import of food and conversation are always a part of the tapestry we call hospitality.

It is important to acknowledge that food and drink are critical elements in most religious celebrations, as well. Various forms of Catholicism and Protestant sects have communion and wine as focal points of their services. Without question, breaking of bread is actual and symbolic in a coming together of spirits.

I know, for me, when I have chance to dine with a new person, the exchange has a much more powerful imprint on me. I have many meetings, but I tend to remember the ones that revolve around food. This might have something to do with my great love of foods, but I think it relates more to the spirituality associated with the moment.

BEING ATTENTIVE TO OTHERS

Another element of hospitality, I've found, revolves around the focus of the exchange. It seems that hospitable people tend to talk less about themselves and want to know more about the person they are engaging. This is not that hospitable people don't have important things to say about themselves; only that they are truly interested in other people. Now this point is important, because many people like to talk about themselves, and to suspend the propensity to do this is not always easy.

It is also important to remember that when asking about others or talking about ourselves we are quick to define ourselves by our vocation or work title. Although this is natural, it can be stunting. When we hear titles or vocations we can easily begin to stereotype people. That is, we discover someone is a banker, we automatically think them to be conservative, or another person is a steelworker we then think them to be hard or macho. We can also tend to either value or devalue people depending on their title. That is, if we feel a certain vocation is more prominent or influential than ours, we will often then defer to them.

When I am invited to speak at conferences, I am intrigued by this "pecking order" mentality. As people self define, the image that emerges at the gathering is interesting to observe. People considered to be less in the translation (less degree, less responsible titles) often seem to be excluded or muted in the conversations I have observed. In practicing our ability to extend to others, we must do our best to suspend discussions in areas that will cause us to stereotype or close down on people.

Counselors know all about this as one key element taught in many schools of counseling is the ability to suspend personal judgement while engaged in counseling activities. Seasoned counselors know this is very difficult to do, but absolutely essential if the counseling is to move forward. To truly make the exchange more successful, the counselor must suspend their judgment. If they harbor a stereotype or judgement about clients they see, the counseling session will be stilted.

I was once invited to a friend of a friend's home for a party. During the course of the evening, I found myself talking with the host for what seemed to be a long period of time. I was considerably at home in the discussion, and found myself truly liking this person. Later though, in reflecting on the way home, I realized that this man talked little of himself and asked more about me.

This is not to say that people shouldn't talk about themselves, or to do so leads to inhospitality. Only that the more one shows an interest in others, the more we learn in the exchange and make people feel good in the translation. This requires the ability to listen.

Now, this notion of listening is a vital ingredient to hospitality. When you pause to truly reflect, the person who listens well is in a direct position to tend to others. As important information is exchanged, the good listener can become more and more hospitable. Others have picked up on this point.

In his observation of servant leadership, Robert Greenleaf (1977) writes about the power of listening:

> a true natural servant automatically responds to any problem by listening first...true listening builds strength in others. (p. 17)

Along with Greenleaf's perspectives on listening and strength we might also add that listening does ignite a fuel for hospitality.

It's important to know, too, that listening skills can be developed. People can literally learn to listen better. One method that can help in this development, is to hold back thoughts and reactions while people are talking to us. In our society, however, this is very difficult to do. Typically, while people are talking to us, we are usually half listening, half formulating our response. The truly good listener is attempting full concentration on the items discussed. Then after the speaker has concluded, a good listener starts to develop their response.

The next time you are in conversation, why not try this approach. Be totally focused on what the person is saying to you. Then, after they complete their thoughts, pause and formulate your response. This will be awkward at first, but it will truly help in developing better listening skills and that, in turn, will promote a greater feeling of hospitality.

One of the most attentive persons I know, is my friend Jim. He is well-known in our community and well-liked. When I observe Jim in social situations, I am amazed. He relates fluidly and pays deep attention to those he is with. He is a great conversationalist and keeps discussions flowing with detailed questions and inquiry. When I ask Jim about this, he makes no big deal of it. He talks about how interesting people are and how much he learns from his friends. He is an artist in being attentive. Now Jim is not a trained counselor, but he has developed the ability to truly focus and listen to his partner. Think about people like Jim that you know. We could all do more to become better listeners.

BEING UPBEAT

Still another element of hospitality, I think, lies in attitude and affect. That is, the more one seems up and smiles, the more others around them will feel welcomed. There is something infectious about a smile, or nod, or wink of the eye.

To this point, when I enter a room full of new people, I am often engaged by the people who show this type of positive affect. I gravitate to people who are laughing or touching. These physical gestures are hospitable and inviting. I can't tell you the times I'm in a social situation with others and a new person will approach and say they had to join us because we were laughing and affective in our conversation.

This invitation for others to join doesn't just relate to those outward displays of affect. Equally luring are people who show, through their eyes, body language and attentiveness, a true interest in the person or topic. Such an experience again happened to me recently at a conference I presented at in Kansas City. I was conducting a day long workshop on "Culture and Community" to a group of some 75 rehabilitationists. As I moved about the room raising questions and focusing the discussion I was caught be a woman sitting off to the side. Even though she participated no more or less than the others in the workshop I felt a presence, energy, and interest from her. Later, after the session I bumped into her at a conference reception. Once we began to talk the connection was immediate and before too long we were deep in conversation. Her perspectives and upbeat nature was truly delightful, and now my friend Chris and I correspond regularly.

I have many friends who practice this positive affect to a tee, but my friend Ralph is a magician at being upbeat. I see Ralph often as our children go to school together and I can never recall not seeing him smile. This is not to say that Ralph doesn't have his bad moments; I'm sure he does. It's more that he has an attitude for life that is solid and warm. Folks like Ralph, have a natural affinity for life and draw people toward them. When I think about Ralph and others with similar dispositions, I observe some common themes. They smile a lot, and always have a positive word. They find good in people and relate to all different types of folks. Some people tell me that such an affinity is a gift, but I seem to think that this gift can be developed. To do so, however, requires a conscious and concerted effort.

I talked to Ralph about his positive outlook and his response was typical to most upbeat people I know. He talked about how fast life seems to go and how futile it is to mope. He said that when he finds himself getting down, or he is reminded by his wife Sandy that his mood is turning sour, he tries to consciously shift gears; to reflect on the good things around him and how fortunate he is to have them.

This is a simple conclusion, one I am sure you have thought about, yet my friend Ralph is truly on to our important element. To be up in spirit is a process that often requires a conscious and direct effort. Like Ralph, many of us need to develop a trigger that can push us to being up, because when we are, the route to hospitality becomes that much easier.

EXTENDING TO OTHERS

Continuing in this laundry list of elements that relate to hospitality is the basic notion of extending out to others. This is found when we make a conscious effort to include or welcome others into our presence. Again, I am called to my observations of yet another relative, a true purveyor of hospitality, Aunt Dolly.

My Aunt Dolly and Uncle Mus are really unique people. Any student of hospitality would do well to spend time around them. First, it is important to know that Aunt Dolly and Uncle Mus are in-law relatives, the sister and brother-in-law of my wife's mother, Concetta. (You remember Coungy – she serves as a mentor in kindness.).

For as long as I have known my wife, some 29 years, Aunt Dolly and Uncle Mus have been a constant source of welcome and openness. They live in the Washington, DC area, and over the years, the Fallon (their last name) motel, as we call it, has been home for my DC trips. There are many stories of hospitality from the Fallon homestead, but one that sticks out most happened in 1973. I remember the year because I was doing military duty at the time and our summer camp that year was at Fort AP Hill in Northern Virginia. It was a hot camp that year, and over the weekend, five friends and I got a pass. With only a few hours, and less money, we were thinking about what we might do. On a whim, I suggested we go up to DC and visit Aunt Dolly and Uncle Mus. They had a pool in the back yard and we could cool out there.

Trying to be considerate, I called them up but the line was busy. Since we didn't have much time, and I knew they were home I suggested we go, even though I couldn't reach them. In due time, we arrived in Alexandria and six hot soldiers stood on their porch as the doorbell rang. When Aunt Dolly opened the door, she didn't miss a beat. With a hug and a smile, she opened the door and her home to us. We swam, Uncle Mus cooked up some hot dogs, and we relaxed by their pool.

Later, while driving back to Fort AP Hill, my friends were marveling at how great Aunt Dolly and Uncle Mus were, I mentioned that all of my wife's relatives are warm people. My friend, Bruce, said, "Wait a minute, Aunt Dolly and Uncle Mus aren't your blood relatives?" I told him that we were related through marriage and the car fell silent. Needless to say, these fellows could not believe that a family could be so welcoming, especially to an in-law. None of my friends, that day, could fathom calling on relatives, the way we did, let alone non-blood relatives. Such is the way with Aunt Dolly and Uncle Mus.

One more point, while we're on this topic of extending out to people. A number of years ago, through observing a good friend, I learned another subtle, yet important aspect about hospitality. I see this friend at conference gatherings a couple times a year when our schedules trail together and he is truly a hospitable man. As a student of hospitality, I have been studying his style, and I notice that Kenny always extends himself to others. For example, if we're standing in a small circle at a gathering, and a new person approaches, Kenny always is conscious to welcome the new person, make a space for them, introduce them, and then fill them in on the conversation to that point. It is a simple gesture, but he never fails to do it.

I am struck by this because it is a basic act of hospitality, yet think how infrequently it happens. The typical scenario is that the new person must wait until the conversation kicks to a new topic and then they can jump in. It's almost as if the new person must pay some dues until they can join the group. All of us know how awkward it might be to mingle at gatherings, still we fail to do a basic act of hospitality that would make this hurdle easier to handle.

FURTHER PERSPECTIVES ON HOSPITALITY

I asked my dad about his thoughts on this topic; how he came about his gift of hospitality. After reflecting for a minute, he told me about a custom they had in his home as a young boy. If he or his brothers or sisters were called by any elder, rather than say "what" or "yes," they had to respond "Chi command." This is an Italian phrase that means "who commands me." These are interesting words as they imply that the responder is at the commandment of the person making the request. This gesture validates and enhances the value of the person making the request.

Another custom was to never expect, or even allow, the guest to ask for something in their home. Rather, the host would regularly inquire if the guest was all right, if they needed more coffee or food. It is a measure of anticipation that is prevalent throughout all of the Condeluci households. This custom is intriguing because it suggests that the host put himself in the guest's place— sort of how it would feel if the tables were reverse.

Now, I'm not sure, as is my dad, that these customs alone are responsible for creating a sense of hospitality. Obviously, there are many factors that have converged in my dad's life to build the man he is. Still, these notions of "who commands me" or being anticipatory are key starting points to interchange; and, hospitality has to start somewhere.

I talked too, with my mother to glean her early notions of hospitality. She remembered warmly the atmosphere in her home as a young child, where others were welcomed with food and drink. In fact, mom said that the feelings were so welcoming that early the next morning, long after the guests departed, she and her sisters and brother would slip downstairs and consume the remains of the food. To her, the thoughts of visitors to their home lived on, even to the next day. I pushed mom in my inquiry to give me, in a few words, a definition of hospitality. After a few moments, she said, "When you treat others as your own."

Think about this – treating others as your own. It's a simple point, yet hard to actualize. It is a perfect "momism." So often, when we meet new people, there is that awkward period when we make small talk and try to get to know the new person. At this juncture in the interchange, are we looking for points of commonality or of difference?

It's my sense, at this phase, we should be looking for points of commonality. When this happens, I am sure we will find that the new person will have things about them that are like us. If they are like us then we will be much more quickly engaged by them and willing to incorporate them. If, however, we discover as we talk, that they are very different from us, we are often reluctant to go on with the interchange.

This notion of how we connect with new people will be examined later in this text. It is interesting, and important, though, that the link point of hospitality get us started in the process. If we don't have hospitality as a start point, getting beyond difference will be harder than it already is.

As we think about hospitality, and examine the ways we begin, and then nurture this concept, we must acknowledge the forces that work against hospitality. In some research on this matter, I ran into an interesting thesis by the anthropologist, Edward Hall. In his intriguing book, *Beyond Culture*, Hall (1976) examines the elements that go beyond culture. He suggests that our nervous system was developed long before the speed, pressures, and intensity of current society. He implies that people are better equipped to deal with a slower more public lifestyle where they know those around them and can react to the cues of their neighbors. Of course, in an era when people lived in small tribes or villages, this approach was natural to realize because people knew each other and their patterns. As we think of this propensity in our society today, however, this notion might give us some insights on why it is hard for people to be hospitable to newcomers. In our present society, most people we encounter, even in our own communities get jumbled in our overtaxed, over stimulated world.

Hospitality is about welcoming; it's about opening up oneself to others. All of us know how good it feels to be treated with hospitality and all of us know there is so much more we can do to be welcoming of others in our own lives. We just need to think about it more often and try to do it more regularly.

9

Generosity

*To do something, however small,
to make others happier and better,
is the highest ambition, the most
elevating hope, which can inspire
a human being.*

John Lubbock

9

Generosity

As we move further along this review of key traits getting us beyond difference, next comes generosity. As all the traits we will review can dovetail with each other, the notion of generosity is freestanding as well. It is a word we have all heard before, but for most of us, it is another concept that we don't often reflect on. What does generosity mean to you? What does it take to be a generous person? Can people work to create a greater sense of generosity?

First, a definition of generosity. Consider these from American Heritage Dictionary:

Gen-er-os-i-ty 1. High quality 2a. Liberality in spirit or act 2b. An act or instance of magnanimity or munificence 3. Abundance, copiousness.

Generosity. 1. Readiness or liberality in giving; munificence 2) Freedom from meanness or pettiness, magnanimity 3) Generous act 4) largeness or fullness; amplitude.

It is interesting to note with this definition, the acknowledgment of the spirit. In a way, however, you really can not think of generosity without a solid recognition of the spirit. It seems to be generous is to open the spirit.

I am always taken aback when I meet people who are truly generous, because they seem a minority in today's society. In fact, for some people I know, their basic reaction to generosity is just the opposite of these definitions. It is more of a "Why be generous—what's in it for me?" type of reaction. In this day and age, generosity seems to raise suspicion. People seem to be so into themselves, that someone who freely gives to another raises eyebrows.

It also seems, that when people are uncomfortable with generosity, it can be a sign of their insecurity. It's as if the generous person must be seen suspiciously because the person on the receiving end is not worthy, or will now become beholden. These are sad, but often common conclusions.

This feeling of not being worthy of someone's generosity is, of course, tied to devaluation. When people feel less valued, as people who have difference often do, the ability to accept a gift in an equal, freely given way is compromised. Since the person feels less valuable, they also feel less worthy. It is a spiral trap that is hard to leave.

The other trap, that of becoming beholden, is tied to insecurity and a lack of trust as well. There is clearly a sense in western society, that if you do something for me, then I owe you one. I know many people who keep score of gifts given or received. This cheapens generosity to a game status and clearly perverts the process.

I wonder where this might come from. In my travels, I have asked people their perspective on this very issue of how generosity can be developed or perverted. My friend, Betsy, from Rochester, NY, has a thought on this that is interesting. She contends that the structured social format of our culture, especially that of preschool and kindergarten, sets the stage. In these settings, young malleable children get introduced to, and then positioned and organized around, their "stuff." They have a desk and their crayons, and a special place in the class. They are often taught to guard and tend to their "stuff."

Now surely this initiation to material things that are "owned" can happen well before the school years. Betsy contends, however, that the notion of school where other strangers come together in

less likely to give of fear of view

the first of our formal, common interchange is more imprinting of these things of possession. Of course, the point is that these early experiences then set the course to continue to guard these possessions and keep them safe.

In a broader way, this initial focus on possession seemingly sets the stage for the common American notion that more "things" are better. The more possessions we have and; in an odd way, the bigger they are, then the closer we come to being seen and seeing ourselves as successful. In its further point of perversion, this action leads to the perspective I recently saw on a bumper sticker. It said, "In Life, He Or She With The Most Toys Is The Winner."

Another point for clarification, with this notion of generosity, revolves around the intent of the gift. People can be generous for many reasons. If the generosity is related to some expected result, the purity of the action can be diluted. An example here might be the boss at work giving his employees a Christmas gift. This act of giving might not be generous at all for two reasons. First, it might be given to keep the employee beholden to the boss. Second, Christmas is a traditional time for giving; to a certain extent it is a reason for giving.

We should pause for a moment and reflect on this motive issue. Why do people give? Why do you give? What drives generosity? We all know the Biblical notion that by giving, one will receive far more in return. Yet the Judeo-Christian genesis of this give/receive formula is that people should not give to receive. Still, through giving one gets back far more from the "feeling" of doing good for another person. In the purest sense, there should be no tangible expectations.

Another friend from New York, Janet, suggests that giving is related to passion. She feels that people usually give when they are passionate about someone, or something. That is, when passion is the motive, the bargain of the gift is not necessarily related to what one may receive. The passion of the transaction changes the format of the exchange.

Still, for most people, this sense that there is something in it for me if I give is powerful. It's interesting to speculate where all this comes from. I remember growing up in my large, extended family environment where my brother, sisters, and cousins were prompted to give of our toys and time, to one another. I'm sure, in these early lessons, my parents didn't suggest that through such actions, we would truly reap tangible or even intangible benefits. Only that it was important to share, and be generous with our possessions.

Somewhere, though, the "what's in it for me" attitude crept in. It was at that moment that innocence gave way to calculation, and the true notion of generosity was perverted. I've been curious about this for some time. In my observation of children, I'm always struck by the number of children who easily share with other children. Recently, I was observing my son, Santino's, kindergarten class. Not all the five-year-olds were up to the sharing. Some were, others weren't; but I was amazed how many easily fit in and were generous to each other.

In watching Santino and the other children, I am drawn to that age old question of selfishness and altruism. Clearly, in our world, we know both types of people, but how does all this start? Are we destined to be generous, implanted with some altruistic seed? Or, do we have to balance the natural propensity to be selfish and give only when it best serves us?

My cousin, Dennis, and I have had many a debate about these notions of altruism, selfishness, and generosity. As a biologist Dennis is convinced that actions of generosity are all tied to selfishness. He feels that our main drive is self survival and any generous acts are done to assure our own satisfaction and personal well being.

I, on the other hand, disagree with my cousin. I understand the format of his thesis, but feel he has not factored in the element of free will. I think there are many actions that do not have a tie to self survival. In his book on altruism, Alfie Kohn, (1986) gives example upon example of selfless acts of heroism where there was no identifiable motives, not even self survival.

If we apply some of the concept of generosity to the framework of getting beyond difference, however, we must be able to wrestle first with the "what's in it for me" question. What is in it for us when we apply generosity to the question of difference- when we reach out to be inclusive?

For me, the first answer seems tangible and relatively simple. The result of reaching out to someone who is different from you is the possibility of finding a new and important friend. And most of us could always use new friends. In fact, good friends are hard to come by and the thought of missing the possibility, just because that person is different from you is shortsighted at best.

But I'm not sure this is the case for others. It seems that somewhere in the equation a payoff must fit in for some people. As I innocently ask about this, especially with people in the community, I often find a spiritual conclusion, one that I call the quest for "grace points." What I mean here, is that those who apply generosity to people who are different do so primarily because it earns them "grace points." For these folks the "grace points" are the green stamps to heaven.

Now I don't mean to be cynical here. In fact, I feel that the people in quest of "grace points" are in a better place to get beyond difference than many others; especially those who are caught in hate and avoidance of people who are different. Still, my concern remains. It has more to do with the pity notion of achieving "grace points." People caught in this zone act not from generosity but from pity.

We can consider again, the notion of telethons. Year in and year out, telethons reap millions of dollars for causes that often surround difference. One might infer that the typical telethon donor is generous, and many are. Yet, these donations are often driven by the audience feeling sad and wanting to do something for the telethon recipient. People conversant in telethons, tell me that the more the images pull at the heart strings the more the phones ring with donations.

In spite of some of these realities, I find that another issue to this generosity question is less tangible and clear. Indeed, it is more of a spiritual notion of self discovery. What I mean is that as we reach out in generosity to connect with different people, we are forced to examine our own nature and humanity. In the process of seeking to know someone different, we are really forced to know ourselves. This inward exploration is not easy, but most of the time it is tremendously enriching. It can sharpen our perspectives and allow us to wrestle with the realities, great and small, of our personalities.

For me, then, in this process, there has been an interesting discovery. As I have come to reach out to different people, and then examine my own make-up, I have found that the obvious differences that formerly kept us apart, when compared to the similarities that bond us as people, are minuscule. That after the hurdle is made, the commonality of our wants, needs and desires are indistinguishable. But I had to confront the differences, and generosity is a trait that can bridge that gap.

I remember an experience I had in Europe, a number of years ago, that drove home this point. I was hosting a two week Austrian ski tour sponsored by the travel agency my wife worked for at the time. Europe was new and fascinating, but the obvious differences in language and culture were intimidating to most of us. To this extent, the majority of the members from our party stayed together.

One night, in the village of St. Anton, Austria, a couple of us went out to a local pub, only to find it crowded, with little table space. We were ready to leave when a generous woman, sitting with a group of people, motioned for us to join them, and then squeezed room at the table. As we sat down our smiles gave the message of thanks, but then an awkward silence befell the table. The folks around the table were from many different countries and the languages varied. We were clearly different from one another.

My first attempts to communicate were laborious, but using napkins, pens, and the common bond of skiing, we broke the ice. Before too long, we had learned much about each other. As we pushed into even more complex issues like politics, nuclear proliferation and world events, it became amazing how similar we were.

I often think about this incident, because it was a type of watershed event for me. I remember it as the time I pushed beyond my stereotypes and presumptions into a world of difference only to find myself, and the simplicity of a world commonalty. All because a generous person invited some awkward Americans to join their table.

What is it we have been saying throughout this book — that the smallest, most simplest of experiences are the ones that can count the most. That is why when we open our spirit to other people, we start on the road that can get us beyond difference. All we have to do is take that first step.

Again, my Beyond Difference class conducted in Pittsburgh offered some interesting thoughts about this notion of generosity. When asked to define this concept in a word, the students said,

Generosity is:

to do something	quiet love
giving of self	stretching
sacrifice	total surrender
humility	unselfishness
being humble	faithfulness
no expectations	no motives
from the heart	putting others first
being spontaneous	giving

One student felt that generosity must be immediate and spontaneous. He though that once a person reflects on their actions they become more calculating and this can prevent the action. I think this idea of spontaneity is an important one. Once we hesitate in giving, the spirit behind the gift can get tested and then we can easily drift to another place.

I do know that no matter what route we take, they all start with a consciousness, and then willingness to be more generous. We must think about others and the importance of giving. I was recently in Little Rock, Arkansas to participate in a conference. After the sessions concluded, I was sitting around with some friends and we were talking about this notion of generosity. Most people concluded that the tone for generosity was set with early experiences with family, however, it was also acknowledged that somewhere in the scheme of growing up, a more selfish agenda occurs. Some of those in the conversation, felt that the natural tendencies of egocentricity take over. Others felt that the rigors of competition push people toward selfishness.

I'm not exactly sure where I stand on this issue. I do agree that there is a hiatus in generosity as we grow, that people do get side-tracked from the lessons of our youth. Of course, some of us never get the early lessons in the first place as families are caught in the spiral of today's pace. I'm fearful that this is happening more today than ever. Countless children are in family situations where only one parent is present, or where both parents are just too busy. In these situations, the lessons of generosity may get compromised, or may not be happening at all.

I am certain that the competitive spirit of our society also has an impact. It's pretty hard to be generous, when the rules of the game suggest that you win at any cost. It's important to acknowledge that this competitiveness is not just a factor of sports. Our schools, clubs and social institutions all promote a sense of competition that may stunt generosity.

I'm intrigued too, by the competitive notion that tangibilizes actions. There seems to be some unwritten law of our culture that says each thing that I give is less I have. In this analysis, if the rules of the game are to have more, as the bumper sticker says, "He with the most toys wins," then to give anything away is a detriment. This gets to be so strong of a notion that it applies to others things as well, like the benefit of the doubt.

Alfie Kohn (1986), again, has done some interesting study and writing on the issue of competition. He concluded that all types of competition, even the so-called "healthy competition," is destructive to people. Instead, in his work, he promotes the notion of co-operation. He states:

> Researchers have shown repeatedly that cooperation pre-dicts to learning more than does competition or individu-alized attainment. It's true in rural, urban, and suburban schools; it's true for all ages; it's true for all subject matters. And the more complicated the task is, the worse competi-tion does; the more cognitive problem-solving and creativ-ity is required, the worse competition stacks up when mea-sured against cooperative approaches. (p. 14)

As I continue to think about generosity, or more importantly, the things that develop or stunt this trait, I am drawn to more closely examine our educational methods in western culture. Recently, I explored the educational paradigm, using some of Paulo Freier's thesis. In his work, *Pedegogy of the Oppressed,* Freire (1989) reviews the key tenants of the "banking" method of education. He states:

+ The teacher teaches and the students are taught
+ The teacher knows everything and the student knows nothing;
+ The teacher thinks and the students are thought about:
+ The teacher talks, the students listen – meekly;
+ The teacher disciplines and the students are disciplined;
+ The teacher chooses and enforces his choice, and the stu-dents comply;
+ The teacher acts, and the students have the illusion of acting through the actions of the teacher;
+ The teacher chooses the program content, and the students adapt to it;
+ The teacher confuses the authority of knowledge with his own personal authority, which he sets in opposition to the freedom of the students;
+ The teacher is the subject of the learning process, while the students are mere objects.

Although Freire's outline is stark, for most of us in western cultural situations, we can find reality in every indicator he has identified. As I think about this, the notion of the parameters and control to what children learn and adapt to can set a powerful tone. This is not to say that every element of student exposure to this paradigm will be limiting or problematic, but clearly can be skewed.

Using Freire's analysis, and looking around at current elements of our culture, it is easy to see how generosity can be stunted or dismissed. The dimensions identified by Freire can polarize students, bait competition, and promote a situation where there are winners and losers. In a society where the theme is to take, be suspicious and to look out for oneself, learning to be generous can be difficult to do. Given these realities, we must hunt for conscious examples of ways to be generous. We must dig for stories or experiences where people step beyond selfishness to freely give to others.

Now Freire is not the only thinker that has found some of the narrowness of our educational experience. Anthropologists and sociologists have also identified some of the confining nature of education. This narrowness can then lead to a skewed perspective on generosity. Edward Hall, again, in his book, *Beyond Culture* (1976), points out how culture has created some illusions about education. He states:

> Public and private education is another example of the lengths to which extension theory distortions can go. Not only children but people of all ages have the capacity to learn naturally. What is more, learning can be its own reward...Yet the process has been distorted in the minds of the educators, who have confused what they call education with learning. The popular notion is that the schools contain the learning and their job is somehow to get the learning into the child...Modern education has left us with the illusion that a lot is known about learning, that real learning goes on in the school, and that if it does not happen under the aegis of a school, it has no validity. (p. 35)

This thesis about education is important to the question of generosity for a number of reasons. One, is that the schools host children who are easily influenced. In most public education situations, facts and figures are promoted, and the more intangible notions of kindness, generosity, and cooperation get lost in the translation. Most secular schools just stick to the facts, are primarily homogeneous and stress great competition between the children. Indeed, today, some 45 years after the segregation lawsuit Brown vs. Topeka, public schools are more segregated by race and economics than ever before. These influences set strong tones that can affect or even thwart a sense of openness or the promotion of generosity. Take, for example, a situation where testing occurs. The challenge imposed on children is not just to do well, but to do better than your peers. Often, in these types of scenarios, there is little room for the spiritual traits examined in this book. The goal is measured by the child's place in the academic or athletic pecking order, not by thee content of their character.

Tied to education, and equally compromising to generosity, is the dominance of sports in our lives. From the time that children can walk, we begin to influence their reality through sports. Quickly, the fun of sports give way to the pressure of winning. Most people reading this passage can remember or have observed the perversion in sports to the focus of winning. The more noble notion that playing the game well has all but lost out to the more primary drive to win at all costs.

Moreover, our society is now pushing the principle beyond winning. Many sports and those with high visibility around those sports are not just satisfied with winning, but must crush their opponent. This reality has reached epidemic proportions. In their book, *The Dehumanization of Man*, Montagu and Matson (1983) explored this notion more than a decade ago. They write about the decivilizing of sport and how it has taken on a warlike reality. They state:

> The psychology of total winning carries implications that are not at all abstract but as plain as the broken nose on an

opponent's face...Winning at any cost means there will in fact be costs, human costs, measured in broken bodies, crushed spirits, and ruined lives. It has been estimated that some 32 college and high school football players are converted into paraplegics every year, that 28 are killed outright, and that no less than 86 of every 100 high school gridders are sidelined for a week or more by injuries. Any boy who plays the game throughout both high school and college stand a 95% chance of a serious injury...It would be difficult to say which is the more victimized child, the physically gifted or the physically inept, by the authoritarian social system of athletically based rewards and punishments. (pp. 203-206)

These data and the present pressure of sports is staggering. Montagu and Matson (1983), none the less, point out that those who lose in sports are branded as losers and carry the weight of the loss on their self esteem. On the other hand, winners are often thrust into a more manic dominance of regimen and practice that lead to a narrowness and limitation of exposure. In the big picture, everyone loses more than they gain. It's also interesting to note that our culture's reaction to the devastation of sport is not to soften the sport, but to make better helmets and pads to lesson the impact of more vigorous blows.

What is meant in the whole of this, is that children who lose, tend to be perceived by others and by themselves as losers. As the winners push forward their drive to win even more, this energy can literally isolate them. Many of us know stories where children who show some athletic promise are pushed to excel in their sport. This means constant practice and attention to their skills. All of this keeps the developing athlete apart from other experience that might balance the student out. The net result of all of this is a narrowness found with most of our elite athletes. Further, it is much more difficult for narrow people to be generous. It seems we need more attention to broadening people, not isolating them.

Consider the 1994 assault on the figure skater, Nancy Kerrigan. The attack was planned and carried out by a rival skater and her entourage. In this case, it is interesting to note that both skaters had devoted most of their lives to their sport. The commentators talked about their dedication and tenacity as athletes when, perhaps, another point could be made about their narrowness caused by years of athletic isolation.

In a larger way, most types of competition, athletic or otherwise, can lead to a distillation of generosity. Some scholars, such as Alfie Kohn, argue:

> In writing *No Contest* (1986), I went through more than 400 studies and slowly came to the position...that competition is destructive and counter productive not merely in excess; it is destructive not merely because we are doing it the wrong way; it is destructive by its very nature. I think the phrase "healthy competition" is a contradiction in terms, and the ideal amount of competition in any environment, the classroom, the workplace, the family, the playing field, is none... After going through hundreds of studies conducted in the classrooms and the workplace, I have become convinced of what I will put in one bold and startling proposition: Not only is competition not required for excellence, it absence is required for excellence... Competition does not promote strong, good individualism. Competition promotes dependency because it requires other people — my self-evaluation is dependent on other people. (pp. 13-15)

Now the works of Kohn and Montague may seem academic until personal experiences hit closer to home. I had such an experience recently. As president of the school PTG where my children attend, I am constantly receiving input or ideas from other parents. Not long ago, a mother called me to voice concern over our schools Athletic Associations guidelines for the Basketball program. To follow this story, you have to appreciate that ours is a small Catholic school, with 300 student enrollment, K through 8th grade. We have few extracurricular activities and basketball is the only sport sponsored by the school.

This parent told me that 19 boys had tried out for the team, and 4 boys, her son included, had been cut. She said that the coach had told her they only had 15 uniforms. Not having much experience with school sports, I couldn't believe that such a decision had been made. I decided to attend the next Athletic Association meeting to voice concern.

At the meeting, I found a roomful of basketball fathers and cheerleader mothers. Halfway through the meeting I raised the question about the "cut policy" and the recent decision. The Athletic Association president started to mention the 15 uniform limitation and I interrupted, telling them that I would be happy to buy 4 more uniforms. "Well, it wasn't just the uniforms, but the coaching time as well." The coach could not effectively spread his time to 19 boys. So I offered to help coach or find another coach. "Well it's more than the coach, but that the facilities aren't large enough," he said. So I offered to help find some practice space that could accommodate 19 boys. "Listen Al," the president finally said, "you just don't understand. We have always had 15 boys, if we add more now we really screw up the works. We accept the 15 best, the others will just have to watch. That's the way life is."

Now there are many things that I do not know or understand, but I did think that a Catholic school basketball program, especially the only team sport in the school, should be more than the 15 best boys. It should be about teamwork, cooperation, learning the game, and fun. It should compliment the lessons learned in the classroom. It should be about inclusion.

When I asked this roomful of Athletic Association parents why it had to be this way, I got blank stares or head shaking that indicated my naiveté. I tried a few other ways to make my case and promote my vision for the basketball program. When it was clear that my points were lost, in desperation, I asked a simple question, one that I believe is appropriate at a Catholic school, "If Jesus was coaching this team, what would he do?"

Silence stagnated the room, people looking awkwardly at each other. Then someone cracked a joke about Jesus having a team of disciples, and the president pushed the meeting to a new issue. There was no further talk about inclusion, exclusion, self-esteem, and participation. Yet, generosity does play a serious role in the notion of inclusion. For people to be included, whether they are people of different cultures, or basketball skills, starts with a basic sense of hospitality and generosity. One must be open in both heart and action to be truly inclusive.

I left that meeting with a resolve to continue to raise the points of inclusion. Certainly, I understand that not all can play, but why can't all be included. In the case of my children's school, is it better to have 19 boys on the team or 15 valued kids on the squad and four "losers" in the stands. What about these four children in the stands? Will they just get over it? Will they become bigger people for the loss? How will they react if they get a chance to be on top? What kind of men will they become?

I don't mean to be dramatic, because I know how resilient children can be, but think how better we might become if we didn't have to call on our resilience so often.

Usually, most of us don't think about what is, or should be, important in our lives. We're often caught up in the demands or stresses of life that the important moments and the questions pass us by. Yet, if we're to grow as people or a society, we must find out what is important, and this discovery only occurs when we take time to ponder the questions. What is life about? What is really important in our days? How does generosity relate to all of this?

Now, these are not easy questions. They require that we introspect and this inward examination is revealing. What should we do if we don't like the way we really answer the question? What if we find what really is important doesn't live up to expected standards? So most of us go on our way, oblivious, pushing ourselves away from these moments and if we do ask the questions the standard answers follow. We might say, "It is important to make enough money to provide for my family." Or, "It is important to be a good husband, or a good citizen, or to go to church."

But these really just rote answers. They're the ones that most people say, and show no creativity or depth, that we are truly capable of. Indeed, we might as well not answer at all. In fact, I'd contend that the answer to the important question is better nurtured when it sneaks up on us and we realize, hopefully as it's happening, that it is present.

One dimension of this important question happened to me recently and it had taken a real circuitous route. It started simply enough when I decided to take my oldest son, Dante, on a father-son winter Boy Scout outing. Me and my son, in the woods, bonding, as men should do. The intended weekend was free on my calendar, the price was right, and Dante was excited— all the right elements.

We drove the 100 miles to the camp site on a foggy, rainy Friday night. Keep in mind that all of this was new to both of us. As a city kid, I hadn't camped much and Dante's greatest sense of roughing it was a Red Roof Inn with only his "Game Boy" for entertainment.

When we got to the site, we duly registered, got our cabin assignment and our list of activities for the next two days. The perky scout master (there is something about these big boy scouts that make their eyes sparkle) told us to get a good night's sleep because two busy days were in store. He told us that although the snow plans were changed (remember the rain) we would have a great time with Plan B.

As we unloaded the car, Dante and I made sure we brought in our essentials: sleeping gear, Oreo cookies, his portable Nintendo and my work-stuffed brief case. With the bunks made, Dante curled up and being the prepared guy I am, I reviewed the next day's schedule. It spoke of the various competitions, "fire starting, BB guns, log sawing, scavenger hunt, bows and arrows," all the things that are near and dear to my heart; and important things for my son to know?

As night fell deeply to our cabin, we tried to sleep but there is something deadly about giggling 10-year-olds in the next room, a lumpy mattress, and anticipation about "fire starting" competition that forms an irritating gestalt. Needless to say, as morning dawned too soon, we found ourselves up, tired, and the incessant rain falling.

At breakfast I gazed around at a roomful of fathers and sons, 100 in all. Some were big, others small, all shades of color and background. As we stood for the first formation I wondered about these men. Why were we there?

Our first event was the ever popular fire starting contest. Each father-son team was asked to fetch wood and kindling and bring it to an area marked off by stakes and two strings, one 6 inches from the ground, the other 12 inches from the ground. Along this course there were 12 inch wide stations and each team was designated to a station.

As we stood in the rain, getting our instructions from another upbeat scout master, I couldn't help notice that the dad on the team to our left had a ball cap and warm up jacket proudly displaying the sign "Renderdale Volunteer Fire Co." and the name "Tommy" on the left breast pocket. "Great, a damn fireman, just my luck," I thought.

Instructions rendered, the scout master looked at the stopwatch and said "go." Fathers and sons scattered. Dante looked at me and said, "What should we do, Dad?" Innocent question sure, but the logic of the whole thing didn't fit well for me. This is not to mention the rain that made the scene even more bizarre.

I looked blankly to my right and a few stations away was a man from my cabin, a slight fellow relatively new to the United States from New Delhi. Our pained eye contact was both pitiful and pleasing. Pleasing in that I knew I wasn't alone, but pitiful that in his case, he could use the newcomer status as an excuse — I could not.

Finally, I said to Dante, "Well, let's get some wood and see if we can get a fire started." I hadn't finished my sentence when Tommy,

the Renderdale pyromaniac, was back with his boy and already setting the base for his fire.

Dante and I stumbled around in the weeds. There wasn't a dry
twig to be found. Undaunted, however, we gathered some wet wood
and returned to our station.

By this time, Tommy was on the ground blowing into a heaped
concoction that was spilling out smoke. I was sure he had some
gizmo from the fire station making his fire happen.

The scout master, noting the vast discrepancy just between our
two stations took pity on us and passed Dante a few wooden matches.
Still, we couldn't get it started.

In record time, Tommy burned both strings and won thee competition. In a veiled effort to push sportsmanship over victory, the
scout master told the rest of us to continue with our fires. Then, in
a smart-ass manner Tommy looked at me and said, "Take a few of
my embers maybe you can start your fire with them."

A lesser man would have yielded, but we didn't need Tommy's
help. Dante and I struggled onward, but to no avail. The rain and
our ineptness were the victors. Dante suggested I take Tommy's
embers, but I'd have none of that.

Thankfully time ran out, and the scout master declared Tommy
and his son the winners. As we sloshed onward toward our next
event, I struggled to find a way to make this fit for Dante. I was
ready to offer him the standard cliches, "We did our best" or "at
least we tried," when Dante looked at me and said, "This is neat,
isn't it Dad?"

A thousand rocks falling on my head couldn't have been more
stunning. Our eyes locked and then I realized it really didn't matter
if we won, or even got it together to find a dry twig. What mattered
to Dante was that we were together, trying something, working to
figure out a challenge. Two men together, alone in the midst of a
hundred, solving a problem. The reality was complex, yet simple.
The competition was my baggage, not Dante's. What was important to him was being with me, not that we won.

I stopped walking and looked intently at Dante; the specks of rain on his face. For that moment, we were bonded, blended together in the spirit of one. His innocence blinded me. Seconds seemed like an hour. The real student in the situation was me.

Although these stories drive home the points related to generosity and competition, the good news is that somewhere down the road many of us resurrect the notion of generosity. Those basic experiences and instincts of our youth push back into our consciousness and the "what's in it for me" attitude for some can drift away.

This too, is hard to scientifically predict or promote, but it seems to happen to people in different ways. Sometimes it's insidious; other times it might be very stark. Regardless, it's great for us as a collection of people when it happens. When generosity happens, it makes us better as people and as a society.

With both the insidious, as well as stark examples of generosity reborn, it seems that a type of maturation is at the core. People somehow begin to touch their own mortality and when they do the potential for generosity grows. That is, as people grow to see that they won't live forever their acts of kindness and generosity become step stones to acknowledgment. These examples are tied more to helping others than helping self.

One clarifying experience for many people is when a friend or loved one dies suddenly. The notion that in a blink of an eye things can change, can be the experience to push people into generosity. I know for me the older I grow, and more wakes I am called to attend, cause me to more often examine my own mortality. This examination then pushes me to think about my actions and behavior with others. It is truly a shame to have delayed an action of generosity only to find those that you care about gone.

In my own observation, it also seems that important relationships are the start point for generosity. Think back to your early experiences. When you first developed an important relationship with someone other than your family, your first inclinations were to give to that person. You wanted to please the person, often times for no reason. Just the look on their face as they receive your gift is often payment enough.

This tie in of love and generosity is legion. Indeed, the whole notion of love, to many who examine it, find generosity inextricably linked. Over the years, many of us have been touched by the writings and words of Leo Buscaglia. His most popular works, *Love* (1972) and *Loving Each Other* (1984), build from the basic premise of love. Buscaglia has a huge following because he touches us at a most basic level.

When you fall in love, or have chance to witness lovers, the flood of generosity is clear. Lovers get lost in each other through their free giving to each other. It's a shame that people don't fall in love (or stay in love for that matter) more. This would surely be a more generous world.

Somehow, and someway, these gestures of generosity to our close relationships can then give way to an even broader perspective of giving. Making the jump from calculated giving, to close relationship giving, to general giving then brings us closer to the basic spiritual notion of generosity. When this happens, you will know it and your life will be more deeply enriched.

I am constantly amazed and touched by acts of generosity that come to me. So often, in the opportunities I have to travel and meet others at conferences, workshops and gathering, people I have recently met reach out with gifts. Sometimes, these are gifts of encouraging words, or thoughtfulness of an idea, or a book or tape.

One such gift was from a warm, generous person I met a few years ago in Toronto Canada. Her name is Eva, and after a presentation I made on the concept of interdependence she approached me to lend a word of thanks. In her own work as a physiotherapist, she often feels oppressed by the medical model and felt that the concept of interdependence would help her stay on track. It is nice to hear these encouraging words, but this day I was down, not feeling that my presentation was really making a difference. We conversed and she helped me focus some thoughts. A few days later, I received a book from Eva titled, *Gifts of the Lotus* (Hawson, 1974).

This small book offers some spiritual thoughts on aspects of the character and of life in general.

I can't begin to tell you how helpful and useful this little book has been. I have read and reflected on its thoughts many, many times. Indeed, I keep the book in my car, and when I come to stop lights in my constant travels around Pittsburgh, I read another passage. Not only has this helped me focus and think, it has also offered solace to an impatient man who would get angry and frustrated when he waits for lights to change.

The book, *Gifts of the Lotus,* was a simple expression of friendship from one person to another, yet it has had lasting impact on me. Not only do the reflections guide me, but it has also linked me to Eva. We write from time to time, and last year, when I had a chance to lecture in Vancouver, she and her husband Rick took me all over that beautiful area of the Pacific Northwest.

We need to keep conscious on the small daily expressions of generosity. The simple truth is that we never know when the next gift will come and the impact it will have on our lives. The beautiful thing is that they come.

I need to tell you about two other gifts given to me, simple yet impactful. One was another book given to me by a new friend named Kerry who lives in Little Rock, Arkansas. After a presentation in that city, Kerry and I were exchanging stories and found that we are kindred spirits. Abruptly, in our conversation he said, "Wait here for a minute, I have something for you." I thought this to be strange because we had just met. Shortly, he returned and handed me, *Life's Little Instruction Book,* by Jackson Brown (1991). I thanked him and then had to rush off for my flight home.

Later that day, waiting for a connection in Charlotte, N.C., I pulled out the Jackson Brown book to read. It was just released at this point and I had no idea of its content or nature. Now, you have to appreciate the scene I was sitting at the gate area, eating some yogurt, when I opened up the book. Brown wrote this book as a gift to his son who was heading off to college. He wanted him to have some thoughts to consider as he moved on his own. The result was some 550 brief items, gentle and kind. I don't know if I was just in one of those sensitive moments, or a tad homesick, but I wasn't even through the introduction when I became sentimental. I thought of my children, and how quickly they are growing. Soon, the tears started to flow. There I was, book in one hand, yogurt in the other, with tears streaming down my cheek. A kindly stewardess, also waiting for the flight, asked if I was OK. These kind of moments are both touching and comic.

The other gift was a cassette tape sent to me by another new friend, Brad. We discovered, during a chat at a conference in Baltimore, that we had similar views, and as we exchanged ideas, I told him about a book I had just read by Ram Dass. He lit up and told me he was a devotee of Dass' work. A few days later, the Ram Dass tape arrived. What a splendid gift. Over and over, when I listen to it, I feel softened and led to even further reflection. You just never know when that next gift will come and how it might affect you.

One important thing about generosity and gifts, especially when the "what's in it for me" phase has passed, is that the gift must always move. I was sensitized to this concept after reading an article of the same name, "The Gift Must Move." I can't even remember the author now, but he contended, and I agree, that gifts are not supposed to be permanent. They are more for the moment and must not be hoarded. Once they have made their impact it is the responsibility of the receiver to move a gift on.

What a wonderful notion! Just think if every gift you received was then passed on to someone else. What a boost to generosity. Rather than give to receive, we receive to give. Such a concept might truly humanize humanity.

As we explore this notion of gifts and generosity, we also must be cautious not to imply that all gifts are tangible or material. Many are, but gifts can come in a number of packages. Probably the strongest example here, is the gift of time. It is often said that the greatest gift is that of time. When you think of this it's true. Most tangible forms of gifts can be replaced. You can always buy another book, or tape you might give to a person, but you can never get back time.

Once it is spent, it is gone. That is why it is so precious, it can't be replaced.

Now this gift of time can not be emphasized enough. In this day and age, we have such demands on our time that life seems to be a blur. We must go here and there, work, family, address home needs, take care of the basics of life. To this extent, when someone takes time to be with us, we must appreciate the importance of this gift.

I was recently in Norfolk, to participate in a conference. As I often try to do when I travel, I called a good friend who now lives in the Virginia Beach area to set up the opportunity to meet. We made our plans, and when I arrived in Norfolk, he met me at the hotel. It was great seeing my friend, Rocky, and we walked around the harbor and talked about many things. As a Christian counselor, Rocky uses spirituality as an important part of his work. It was a great meeting, but what made it even more powerful was that I knew Rocky was making a sacrifice to spend time with me. He has three beautiful children and a wonderful wife. He works hard and as a counselor, spends many nights away from home. Yet, here he was, spending time with me. We wove many thoughts, and I learned much from Rocky, but the real gift to me that night, was his time.

As we reflect on the gift of time, we must acknowledge that some of our western influences can get in the way. Indeed, most people reading these words know that many people subscribe to the notion that time is money. Thus, if your going to give of time, make sure that money, or access to money is part of the bargain. I know people who deeply practice this. Still, the greatest gift is time and when it is given without regard to pay back, it is even greater.

Now most of us need to balance the reality of making a living with the elements of generosity. There is a time for taking and a time for giving. It is important that we know, and practice the difference. Some people might find themselves on either sides of the equation, those that are totally selfless or totally selfish, but most of us fall in the middle. The tract of generosity however, pushes us to think more about the selfless side, where giving is more important than taking.

Recently, in conversation with some folks who present at conferences similar to me, I discovered that a number of people, many who I respect, will not take a speaking engagement unless they are paid a generous fee. Now I don't want to sound like a Pollyanna here, because all of us need to make a living, and I don't really know people's situation. Further, I too, like to be rewarded for some expenditure of time, and if a group that invites me to participate in their gatherings have a budget, I appreciate a fee. But I also know and feel that to be invited to share ideas with groups is an honor and privilege. I also know that some groups do not have access to big budgets. In these cases, there are gifts that must be given.

To a certain extent, time is money and we must respect this. We must not forget, however, that time is also a gift – the most precious that we have, and we must use, and appreciate it this way.

Years ago, when I first started working at UCP, I met a fellow named Don. He is a good person but has some odd manifestations. Most people in the neighborhood steer clear of Don, except for a young fellow named Ken. Ken would regularly visit Don and often they would go out together. At first, I wondered if Ken had some calculated agenda. After some time, however, I realized that it was a solid relationship; Don and Ken truly enjoyed being together, spending time. Both of these men were generous with their time, but in the face of exchange, especially in the era when I met Ken and Don, Ken had so many more options of where and how he could spend his time. Don, on the other hand, given the reality of his devaluation, had much more limited options. In the scheme of things, Ken's hospitality and generosity, especially with his time, was a powerful lesson for me. They are still close friends some twenty years since I first met them.

So how do we promote more generosity? We know the good that a society can do. We also know some of the reasons why generosity is so hard to teach or to come by. We live in a fast paced, highly competitive world. We may not be able to change these realities, but we can look for the high points.

The major route to generosity is through consciousness, and alertness to the many ways and opportunities to give to others. We can do this through our time, money, talent, or teaching. Indeed, perhaps the greatest contribution we can make in promoting generosity is to teach those on our watch of the importance of gift giving. We have opportunities daily to share these notions with others. Let's not miss any more chances.

10

Compassion

Compassion is the basis of
all morality.
                Arthur Schopenhauer

10

Compassion

Continuing on the odyssey of traits found to be instrumental to getting beyond difference, one of the most intense, is compassion. We hear of compassion and surely consider some people we know to be compassionate, but what about this trait is real to you? Compassion is defined by American Heritage Dictionary as:

Com-pas-sion: A deep feeling for and understanding of misery or suffering and the concomitant desire to promote its alleviation: spiritual consciousness of the personal tragedy of another or others and selfless tenderness toward it. *Compassion:* A feeling of deep sympathy and sorrow for someone struck by misfortune, accompanied by a desire to alleviate the suffering; mercy.

When I looked and then reflected on these definitions, two words jumped out at me — selfless and tenderness. What a warm and wonderful notion these words create. A selfless tenderness toward the tragedy of others. Wouldn't any of us, in the face of personal adversity, want someone with us who has a selfless tenderness toward our situation? Indeed we would, and so we have, I believe, the essence of this notion of compassion.

Although one can find solid reference to compassion in the literature, one spiritualist who has become closely associated with compassion is Ram Dass. His journey has been an interesting one.

Back in the early 60s, Dass was known as Richard Alpert and was on faculty at Harvard University. As a colleague of Timothy Leary, Dr. Alpert was a psychologist interested in ways to alter the consciousness. Together, Leary and Alpert experimented with mind-altering drugs and their actions led way to expulsion from Harvard.

As Leary spiraled further to the fringe, Alpert decided to go East and explore mind-alteration in another way. His own state of consciousness made for a vulnerable student. In India, he met his Guru, Maharaj-ji, and began a whole new direction. After years of study, he was given the name, Ram Dass and instructed to go back to the West to teach and live compassion. His writings, *Be Here Now* (1972), *Grist for the Mill* (1976), *How Can I Help* (1985), and *Compassion in Action* (Dass, & Bush, 1991) are all expose's on this notion of compassion. Here are some of Dass' conceptualizations of compassion:

> When you have the compassion that comes from understanding how it is, you don't lay a trip on anybody else as to how they ought to be....Compassion, simply stated, is leaving people alone. You don't lay trips. (1976)

> Compassion is the tender opening of our hearts to pain and suffering...It is working with others in a selfless way, in a spirit of mutual respect. (1991)

> Compassion actually means 'suffering with.' We are looking for ways to help and yearning for growth in ourselves, and we often find both of these in community in the presence of others. The spiritual journey is more of one of listening and tuning to what is...than of choosing...it is a progression from truth to ever deepening truth. (1991)

> Compassionate action is a continual process, one of discovering ever new questions rather than answers. (1991)

Compassionate action is not done for others, it is done with others, for ourselves because we can no longer avoid it. It helps fulfill our lives. (1991)

These passages set some interesting tone to understanding compassion. Dass acknowledges the fact that compassion requires a tender opening of the heart. This reference to tenderness is, I believe, an important one. Dass suggests that the compassionate person is one who is not only tender, but gentle in manner and action.

I'm engaged by this aspect of tenderness. When we see or experience a tender moment, it often can get etched into our memories. It seems that in this day and age, when haste and speed are the premium, tenderness is somewhat out of place. How does tenderness actually look? How can we be more tender? Should we only reserve our tender moments for our loved ones, or our babies? Wouldn't it be a better world if more people were tender with each other?

When I observe tender acts, especially between people who might not be quickly associated with tenderness, I am always touched. To see old friends meet up after a long lapse of time, to touch and revere in each other can bring a tear to the eye. Indeed, Madison Avenue knows well the power of tender moments and when a product can be positioned in the middle, a powerful result can occur.

Remember back a few years ago, to the now classic Coca Cola commercial with football great, "Mean Joe Greene." As the story goes, Joe Greene is heading into the locker room after what appears to have been a brutal football game. He is limping, clearly in pain, and sweating profusely. Halfway down the runway, a young boy offers Joe a drink of his Coke. First, Joe shrugs him off, but the child persists, saying, "It's OK Joe, go ahead, have some." Finally, Joe relents, drinks down all the Coke and shuffles off without acknowledgment. The boy turns sadly to head out the other way then he hears, "Hey kid – here," and he tosses him the game jersey with a warm smile. The boy's face glows and every person watching the commercial is touched by the tenderness of the moment.

The power of this type of commercial is an exposé on compassion. The boy sees Joe's suffering and acts by offering the Coke. Joe accepts, but then just seemingly walks out on the boy's kind act. Just when the boy begins to suffer, Joe acts compassionately by tossing his shirt over. Two acts of compassion that make this commercial a true winner.

Other commercials, many produced for Hallmark cards or ATT, show compassionate acts or calls that are touching. In fact, most tender exchanges we see in advertisements or movies are interesting portrayals of compassion. We do well to study them and consider ways to add these types of actions to our daily exchanges.

Another point drawn by Dass in his writings, relate to the concept of mutual respect. This implies a balance, a partnership between people. When we hold mutual respect for people, we acknowledge our similarities. The notion of mutual respect is, indeed, a key ingredient of interdependence. People who hold a mutual respect for each other understand that they are more alike than different.

Mutual respect is not that easy to carry out for many reasons that we have already examined – competition, societal strata and our propensity to focus on difference. All of these things can interfere with mutual respect and establish some type of artificial barrier between people. The key for me on this point, however, is that you can have difference, strata or competition, and still have mutual respect. We just need to work a little harder at the conscious understanding of the notion of mutual respect. When we shift from what differs us to what we hold as similar, the ability to reach a mutual respect is enhanced.

Throughout most of his work, Dass links compassion to the ability to tune in to others. This ability of tuning is a type of empathy. It suggests a process by which people can get closer to someone's reality. I believe this notion of getting closer to a person's suffering, calls us to think of our own suffering. Earlier in this book, the suggestion was made to recall the times when you were positioned as different. By remembering your own angst, no matter how minor, is a process that helps us to tune in to others.

It is important to differentiate between the notions of empathy, sympathy, and compassion. My friend, Reverend Doctor Bob Miller, helped me understand these themes when he simplified that, sympathy says, "What if he were me?" – empathy says, "There he is." – compassion says, "We're here together."

In this analysis, sympathy centers on self. The person literally perceives the suffering happening to them. I have another friend who can not deal with news reports of suffering because she is so sympathetic to those in need. She breaks down when she sees stories about people starving or being oppressed. In these examples, sympathy can be dysfunctional.

Empathy, on the other hand, centers on the other. It is the ability to focus on the suffering others might be going through. Empathy is often said to be the ability to walk in someone else's shoes. Now again, empathy is apart from the suffering. It pulls us to examine the pain and to reflect on how it might feel if it were happening to us, but it remains an abstract notion. It lingers outside of us.

Compassion, however, differs from sympathy or empathy because it denotes an action of being with the person who suffers. Not only is it action oriented, but some suggest that compassion demands a sense of confrontation to the oppression with those who suffer. In some ways, compassion is a type of solidarity with the hurting person.

This implication of being with others, in a type of solidarity, is also about displacement of the compassionate person. That is, as the compassionate person moves to be with those that suffer, they often must move from a position of privilege to the level of those who suffer. This displacement can put the compassionate person at serious risk. For example, when someone like Ghandi went to support people who were suffering he was at the same risk as those he joined. Others, like Dr. Martin Luther King, lost their lives when they positioned themselves side by side those that suffer. This notion of displacement is an important variable in understanding compassion.

Scholars who have written about compassion, or any of the other traits examined in this book, speak to the fact that becoming compassionate is a process; it is something that we must work at. In some regards, the more compassionate we are, the deeper we grow in understanding compassion. Dass says compassion is about discovering questions rather than finding answers. This inward exploration of self then helps us to more fully reach out to others.

Similarly, the emphasis of compassion is not about achievement, but about what we receive from each other. People who are truly compassionate are not worried about their own glory or accolades. Indeed, the selflessness of compassion is focused on others.

A final point revealed in Dass' definitions of compassion, is that in compassion, we are not reaching out to help, but to be with others. He says that compassion is not done for people, but with them. This is an important theme, because compassion is not about pity. Although it acknowledges suffering of others, it does not suggest that the compassionate person has pity for those who suffer.

Earlier in this book, we looked at the notion of pity as it relates to difference. It might be a good pause here to review that section. Pity is a downward phenomena, one where a person feels sorry for another. It implies a difference between the players. With compassion, we are looking at being with people in mutual respect. There is clearly a difference. Dass (1985) stated, "Compassion is the spontaneous response of love; pity, the involuntary reflex of fear."

Same too, is that compassion is not about charity. The compassionate person is not acting as they do because they are charitable. In fact, charity, like pity, can be more of a downward action, a type of give-away to those less fortunate. In today's context, charity is not about mutual respect. Rather, charity is an action that can be attributed to a society when people are fully compassionate.

I was recently at a dinner party with some friends and I asked about compassion. I wondered how they defined this concept; who was the most compassionate person they knew. My friends, by and large, defined compassion as a willingness to do things for people, especially when they are down and out. One suggested that compassion was the active state of kindness. I think these perspectives, though common, reveal a dilution to the concept of compassion. As we are not often called to examine compassion and it seems to be an innocent error to think of compassion as doing things for others.

People who have examined and reflected on compassion would challenge my friend's notion of doing things "for" people. The key ingredient again, is to do (or be) "with" the suffering person, not "for" them. Compassion demands an equal action where both parties celebrate and grow through the suffering.

To the question of who they found to be most compassionate, most of my friends named a parent, or a colleague they work with or their spouse. They told stories of how these people would go out of their way to help people out. Many of the examples suggested a selfless nature of the acts. Yet, purists would argue that family bonds or the vow of marriage somewhat oblige the partner to be compassionate. Indeed, when I'm called to identify a compassionate person, of course many people close to my life, similar to my friends, come to mind. Yet, although I respect and love these people, somehow it seems like the category of most compassionate needs to be reserved for the real heavyweights of our time; the hero's of caring.

I remember a few years ago, reading Robert Fulghum's (1990) book, *It Was on Fire When I Laid Down on It.* In his inimitable style, Fulghum tells the story of a photo he keeps on a wall in his office. Every time he looks at it, it upsets him. Still, he is drawn to look at it over and over again. It's a photo of Mother Teresa, and each time he glances at it he feels guilty. The guilt is drawn from the fact that a slight, somewhat frail, elderly woman is, single-handedly, changing the world. Day in and day out, she puts her compassion out there on the line being with those who are dying or suffering. Fulghum knows that compassion can be realized. Mother Teresa is testimony to that. What defies him, is his own shortcomings in being more compassionate himself.

Mother Teresa is one of those "caring heros." So is Jimmy Carter, Nelson Mandela, and Jean Vanier. And a generation before them, Albert Schweitzer, Eleanor Roosevelt, Ghandi, and so many others. These are true champions of caring. It is not that we don't have hundreds of other unsung compassionate heroes today. We do, and we should all be glad for them. I'm sure you can compile your own list. Still, for someone to live a life of compassion is to show compassion all the time. Most of us have not been able to cut that type of muster, yet interdependence demands we must try. We must think about compassion and challenge ourselves to bring more mutual respect for those who suffer to our everyday lives.

Reverend Doctor Bob also helped me understand that compassion, as it is about the creation of a new life of equality, is the enemy of competition. That is, since competition is about the differentiation of our skills or abilities, true equality and mutual respect are hard to come by. Compassion is about gifts and actions that unite, not separate people.

Yet, we all know, and in an earlier part of this book examined, how prevalent and dominant the notion of competition is in our society. We live in a world where so much esteem and reward go to the winners. Consequently, most of us cannot relate to the dimensions of true compassion. We're just too conditioned to be competitive.

Further, true compassion breeds life because it is fulfilling. It is a celebration of activity and reaffirms life through mutual respect. That is, although the compassionate person spends the majority of their time with those that suffer or are underprivileged, it is not necessarily somber time. Just being with people is the fulfillment of human destiny.

Now this notion of fulfillment and celebration in addressing suffering is a hard concept for most of us Westerners to understand. We are so conditioned to see suffering and wounds from a perspective of sadness that the idea of mutual respect and fulfillment seem alien. Yet, in a holistic way, action with those that suffer can be fulfilling, but it takes a change in our own perspective.

COMPASSION 175

So, if compassion is a trait that only few aspire to, why spend time exploring it? The answer to this question is simple, because all of us can get further on the compassion continuum. Since compassion is a means, rather that an end, we can all incorporate compassion more into our lifestyle; but it only happens when we think, reflect, and then act on this concept.

Stop now, and reflect. How can we be "with" people more in mutual respect? How can we confront the "stuff" of oppression and distantiation? How can we be more gentle and tender with others, regardless of where they are in their lives?

These are good questions.

11

Forgiveness

*The weak can never forgive.
Forgiveness is the attribute of
the strong.*

Mahatma Gandhi

11

Forgiveness

As I considered traits that could get us beyond difference, my exploration took me through many spiritual aspects. Most of these spiritual dimensions, the ones articulated in this work, and others that were bypassed, were easy to relate to or discuss. This final one, however, that of forgiveness, was seemingly more difficult to appreciate or understand than all the others. As I thought and read about this dimension, I could understand the struggle that we all have with forgiveness.

In fact, think first about a definition of forgiveness. What does it mean to you? Certainly as children, all of us were introduced to this concept. I remember my mother prodding me to forgive my sister for pushing me down, or to forgive my brother because he didn't know better with some action. Yet, forgiveness is a difficult concept to make happen in our lives. When we look at formal definitions we must examine the root word, *forgive.* Here's what the American Heritage Dictionary says:

For-give 1. To cease to feel resentment against on account of wrong committed 2a. To give up resentment of or claim to requital for 2b. To grant relief from
Forgiveness 1) The act of forgiving or the state of being forgiven; pardon, 2) Willingness to forgive.

Although the words of these definition makes sense, the notion to cease a feeling, or to give up a resentment are very deep and powerful actions to consider. The admonishment, "forgive them" is one we hear all the time. Most of us growing up with some spiritual theology guiding us, found that forgiveness was central. In my Catholic upbringing, we learned that Jesus forgave those who betrayed, persecuted, and then ultimately killed him. Catholic theology admits that forgiveness is difficult, but essential to its practice.

Indeed, all major theologies and their clerics talk about, and many have written about forgiveness. They all contend that we need more forgiveness in our lives and that to forgive is to get closer to divinity. The popular literature also speaks to the intensity and demands that forgiveness brings to the human equation.

In his book, *Forgive and Forget*, Lewis Smedes (1984) says, "Forgiveness is God's invention for coming to terms with a world in which, despite their best intentions, people are unfair to each other and hurt each other deeply." He suggests that forgiveness consists of four stages; the hurt, the hate, the healing, and then the coming together.

Another perspective on the notion of forgiveness, comes from the work of John Roger and Peter McWilliams (1990). These folks have popularized some very basic aspects of life. They suggest that forgiving is just that — FOR GIVING. They state:

When you forgive another, who do you give to? The other? Sometimes. Yourself? Always. To forgive another is being in favor of giving to yourself... The layers of forgiveness, then, are two: first, the person we judged (ourselves or another); and second, ourselves for having judged in the first place. (p. 329)

This angle on forgiveness is almost too simple to seem acceptable. It begs the question, "How can such a simple notion be so hard to carry out?" Roger and McWilliams do acknowledge that when the indiscretion that led way to the judgement is deep or powerful that the healing process does require some time and attention. To this issue of time needed to heal, they suggest:

> If we don't allow ourselves the time and freedom to heal, some of our ability to experience life is frozen — locked away — and unavailable for the "up" experiences we seem to like: happiness, contentment, love, peace. The mechanism that feels the anger and depression is the same that feels peace and love. If you refuse to feel the anger and the pain of the loss (or indiscretion), you will not be able to feel anything else until that area heals...When you open yourself to greater learning about yourself, these areas may "thaw," and the feelings of sadness, fear and anger may surface. If this happens, love yourself enough to go through the healing process you did not allow yourself earlier. You do not need to know what the loss was — it may be a combination of several over many years — you just need to let yourself heal yourself this time. (p. 133.)

In exploration of the notion of forgiveness, my "Beyond Difference" students had some interesting definitions.

Forgiveness is:

faith	being like mom
being able to listen	accepting
letting go	complete understanding
being real	being there
taking a lot	empathy
giving another chance	nurturing
understanding	listening
openness	unconditional love

One student thought there is a clear delineation between apology and forgiveness. One can forgive without an apology, but can not self forgive without the act of apology.

Although these varying perspectives have their unique points, a central theme to this notion of forgiveness wraps around being hurt, and then getting beyond the hurt sufficiently to the point that one can then let go of the pain.

With this basic thread, then we can explore forgiveness within the context of difference. As we do this, I can see both an internal and external application of forgiveness. That is, if I talk about forgivingness to people who have difference, the automatic assumption is that they (the different person) should forgive those who are not different for their indiscretions to the different person. This is one dimension we will explore, but there is an equally powerful external perspective that we must also acknowledge, and this is for the person who is not perceived as different to forgive themselves. That is, I see this dilemma of forgiveness as a two way street. The entire burden should not be on the person with difference, but shared, and equally considered. We must embrace the fact that true forgiveness is that of others and of self. We will explore these throughout this section.

In both regards, it is vital that we embrace the agreed on perspective that forgiveness is terribly hard to do. Smedes (1984) says, "Forgiveness is love's toughest work and love's biggest risk." Most people reading this book would agree.

Recently, I was with some friends on vacation. In fact, I wrote some of this section while at the ocean of the Outer Banks. (It's a shame we can't spend all our time reflecting over the ocean. For me, there is this philosophical splendor about the beach that pushes deeper thinking.) Nonetheless, during that week, I was with friends and while working on this book, used the opportunity to ask people's perspective on forgiveness. Although I had varying details from my friends, most all agreed on the difficulty of forgiveness. My friends felt that the challenge of forgiveness rested with the intensity of the indiscretion. That is, the greater the hurt, the harder the forgiveness. One friend contended that even with the "small" hurts, it was very difficult for her to forgive.

As I think about it, it seems that the more intense the person, the more they are vulnerable to the difficulty of forgiveness. Some people are so acutely sensitive that any indiscretion can cut deep. This is not to suggest that one must be superficial in order to be forgiving – only that intense people must work harder at it. In fact, forgiveness seems to be such a difficult challenge that it pushes any of us.

This notion of intensity is of particular interest to many of us involved in the human services. I'm not sure if its just me, but it seems that an inordinate amount of people I meet in the disability movement have a deep passion and intensity. Perhaps it is the seriousness of our work or the power behind the confines of social injustice. Either way (or both), many people in the human service field would be considered intense. Given some of this tie between the vulnerability of indiscretion for people who display intensity, it might be that many of us are easy marks for a struggle with forgiveness.

THE HURT

In thinking about all of this, it seems that the nature of the "hurt" is an important part of forgiveness. That is, "hurt" can occur at many different levels and in many ways. All of us have had these varying types of experiences. There are times when people consciously and knowingly hurt us. They mean to inflict pain. Think back to times when you have been in an argument with a close friend or family member. As the argument intensified, one of you might have become more personal in the attack, with a clear agenda to hurt the person.

I know a couple who recently split up. As their breakup has proceeded, each of them has become increasingly vicious in dealing with the other. Even though both are wonderful caring people the split up brought out some ugly elements to their behavior. It seems that these type of hurts, the calculated hostile ones, are so much more difficult to forgive.

When we explore forgiveness, in conjunction with difference, sometimes these more calculated types of hurts can be found. A classic example here are the planned indiscretions of whites against African-Americans during the civil rights years. Time after time, there were planned and vicious efforts to physically or psychologically hurt people of color who were only asking for their rights to participate in society. An excellent chronicle of these actions previously mentioned in this text, is found in the powerful tape series, "Eyes on the Prize" (1990). Scene after scene explodes on the screen, as one group of peoples calculate a hurt upon another.

Other groups, too, have experienced the wrath of conscious efforts to attack or hurt people because of their difference. Religious groups, American Indians, Jews, South Africans, and others have been the targets of actions of hate. These are difficult actions to forgive. Indeed, spiritual leaders in all of these causes, ones such as Ghandi or King worked hard to have their followers step beyond the hurt and forgive their oppressors. Some could, others couldn't.

A testimony to how difficult it is to forgive these planned works of hate, is that most of these movements gave birth to other leaders who were more reactionary. People like Malcolm X and Russell Means, had a hard time forgiving people who were directly killing and beating their "brothers." Their suggestion was to fight back – to not accept the indiscretions in a passive way. Mind you, these types of leaders did not suggest premeditated violence (although some in the movements did), but did promote that their people protect themselves from the oppression of others.

Films like "X," "Ghandi," and "Dances with Wolves" chronicle the perceptions and reactions of individuals or groups of people to the actions of indiscretion or hate. The ways some leaders in these movements dealt with and then forgave indiscretions is instructive for us all.

These examples, though dramatic in scope, drive home a powerful message in our exploration of forgiveness. That is, forgiveness is never easy, but when one is faced with conscious, deliberate efforts to hurt, it is even more difficult. When we know people are setting out to hurt us, our family or a group we might be a member of, the cut or hurt deepens.

Another area that is important to consider is hurt caused by unconscious actions. In these cases, we have people who are different subjected to hurtful actions, but the emanation of these actions are not premeditated. Examples here might be when a different person is not included in an activity only because the planners didn't think to ask. Many people make assumptions about others and these assumptions then drive behavior. Often, these assumptions are erroneous, and then hurtful to the individual or group.

I was once with a group of friends at a party. As the night proceeded and people loosened up, a small group I was sitting with started to tease one another. Although there were a number of people who had disabilities in the circle, one fellow, because of cerebral palsy, had a speech impediment. The teasing was going on and he ribbed me about something. My response was to rib him back, but in doing so, I mimicked his speech. Immediately, I could tell that I hit a sensitive cord. Although I didn't mean to, I had really hurt him with my behavior.

Immediately, I apologized. He forgave me, and then proceeded to tell me that he never expected me, a person he deeply respects, to make fun of his speech. This experience was both a lesson in forgiveness and behavior for me. You never know when your actions might be misconstrued or perceived as hurtful.

This notion of interpretation is an important concept to factor in when thinking about forgiveness. In simple terms, one can only hurt in conversation if their words are designed, or misinterpreted as mean. That is, in some instances the things we say are designed to hurt. At other times, our words are misinterpreted and then perceived by the receiving party as hurtful. In these examples, the hurt can be just as intense, even if it was not intended. In fact, nonintended, but hurtful words that are misinterpreted, can hurt all the more.

I was at a management seminar this past year and a key point that the facilitators presented was that so many examples of mediocrity in business are related to the interpretation factor. They suggested that we all have a semantic script in our heads that guide our interpretation of messages. This notion of interpretation is important to consider in what hurts us and who we forgive.

In some regard, the growing amount of sexual harassment in the work place can be related to the interpretation factor. As women move toward full acceptance and equality some men in the work place just don't get it. Their mental script sees women as sex objects, things to be pressured, and they believe this is what women want. To a large extent, the Anita Hill – Clarence Thomas affair of 1991, was a conflict of interpretation. Although there was denial playing out, these two people clearly had a different interpretation of the actions.

Some of the more classic examples of unconscious hurtful actions are found when people are subjected to conditioned behaviors. In the southern part of the United States, for example, during the civil rights years, many people participated in hurtful action, but did so only because they were following conditioned practices. This is not to say that these behaviors were right, only that they were conditioned actions from years and years of business, as usual.

These unconscious indiscretions are the most complex when we consider hurtful actions applied to people who are different. There are many reasons for this. One is tied to the deep social wound experienced by people whose difference has been ostracized. Many of my friends with physical disabilities tell me how vulnerable they feel because people have just not taken the time or energy to know them as people. When you have these experiences, over and over, the wound cuts deep. Then the reactions, or in some cases overreaction can be intense. It's easy to interpret the words (or misinterpret) when you have been treated in an ostracizing way. Time and again, people with difference experience behavior that is conditioned and hurtful.

Consider these:

+ The person with AIDS who is totally excluded because some people think that mere presence will result in infection of others.
+ The person with cancer, whose friends abandon him because they think he would rather be alone with his illness.
+ The person with a disability who is not hired for a job because the employer thinks co-workers will make fun of them.
+ The African-American shopper who is followed around the store because he is seen as a threat to steal merchandise.

All of these examples are hurtful, demeaning, stereotypic, or compromising. Indeed, the disability example is illegal given the Americans with Disabilities Act (PL 101-336). Still they happen.

They are also complex because they can confuse, or even compromise, the issue of forgiveness, with education, and legality. That is, what should the person with difference do in these instances? Forgive, educate, or sue?

Recently, at a presentation at Virginia's Woodrow Wilson Rehabilitation Center, exploring the five traits, a student asked me if you had to forget the hurt to truly forgive. This is an interesting concept to ponder. As I see it, some hurt can be forgiven and forgotten — others can be forgiven and never forgotten. That is, it seems to be the residue of the act and not necessarily the act itself that is the core of forgiveness. If someone levies a hurt on me, I might never forget that the action occurred, but still can forgive the action itself. Indeed, some who have thought about forgiveness in a deeper way than I suggest that forgetting the hurt might tend to repress the event only to allow its resurfacing at a later time. This is evidenced by people who have repressed sexual abuse, only to have the ugliness rear its head later in life through perverse or abhorrent behavior.

I have some friends with disabilities who have forgiven so much that they too, have become conditioned to the indiscretions. That is, their forgiveness has transformed their behavior to acceptance, and in turn, have not advanced society to change in any major way.

I opened my book, *Interdependence*, with a story about how two friends and I were refused service in a bar in Harrisburg PA., primarily because my friends had obvious disabilities and the bartender felt they shouldn't be served. As one fellow in our party, Tom, became irate and passionate about the discrimination, my other friend, Harry, suggested we back off and leave the bar. Harry has been in many situations where indiscretions have occurred and he has grown to be quite content to just walk away. It may, in fact, be forgiveness to a fault.

This raises an important question, "Can we be too forgiving?" Can we let people off the hook when, indeed, they should be taken to task? Is Harry too easy on people who should be redirected? These are not easy questions. We often say, "to err is human, to forgive is divine." Is there a limit or threshold to forgiveness that we can't get beyond?

To this extent, forgiveness must be considered in a broader context. It plays a role in dealing with difference, but must be extended if we are to get beyond difference. This extension relates to the role forgiveness plays in everyone's lives. It seems that things related to difference, be they physical, cognitive, spiritual or racial, won't happen until forgiveness happens on the other side of the equation. That is, inclusion for all people in our society must require that we everyday people forgive ourselves for the limitations placed on ourselves and the wrong we do to others.

In this way, forgiveness can be our liberation to get beyond difference. Forgiveness from our past indiscretions and then an awakening to the bond of our similarities, is truly the stepping stones to inclusion. Know, however, that this is a spiritual notion and not easily achieved. As hard as it is to forgive others, so too, is it challenging to forgive ourselves. Yet, this is a critical step to change.

FORGIVENESS AND HATE

If you follow Lewis Smedes stages of forgiveness, after the hurt phase, is hate. Hate poses a curious agenda when you think about self forgiving. It is easy to follow the Smedes stages in the notion of forgiveness of others, and especially if the person who posed the hurt did so consciously. It seems logical that if the hurt is great enough, hate will follow. With conditioned behavior, hate has a more evasive target. That is, do you hate the person who does something to you, or the general attitude about your difference that has driven the behavior? Further, if you are on the other side of difference, how do you even know when you are part of the wounding?

I was once out for dinner with my friend, Judy, who uses a wheelchair and when we went to order at a restaurant, the waitress posed the question of her selection to me, as if she couldn't order for herself. Judy softly corrected the waitress and then said to me, "I hate when service people do this to me."

In this example, Judy forgave the waitress, but has a problem forgiving the general attitude that people with disabilities are helpless. But what about the waitress, how will she know that she "hurt" my friend through her behavior? She probably walked away from the experience with no reflection at all. I suppose that if she thought about her behavior, was attuned to her action, she might feel some remorse. This consciousness raising must be part and parcel to the beyond difference thesis. That is why this section is looking at five vital traits and that forgiveness must happen in concert with the other four.

SELF-FORGIVENESS

Still, the notion of self forgiving continues. Smedes says, "The pain we cause other people becomes the hate we feel for ourselves for having done the wrong." When the waitress feels the pain she caused to my friend, however slight, then she is ready for self forgiveness. But how do we get to this point? What is our responsibility to sensitize or educate people who cause veiled hurts?

Certainly, the organized approaches to difference, the ones we explored in the first section, have the education/sensitization agenda on their docket. To this cause, there are many good works of advocacy and education that are helpful. Indeed, I am planning a follow-up book to this one that looks at external strategies for change. Our call, at this point however, is to raise the consciousness of spiritual traits necessary to get beyond difference.

Once people are aware of their indiscretions, as with any of us who are awaken to change, Smedes calls for the following actions:

First, to be honest with ourselves.
Next, to clear our heads to make way for a forgiving heart.
Third, to be courageous; forgiving is love's ultimate daring.
Fourth, to be concrete with yourself.
Last, to confirm self-forgiveness with the act of love.

Are these steps easy? No! But they do offer a formula to incorporate forgiveness into our strategy base to get beyond difference.

A final point on self forgiveness comes from David Schell (1990), in his book, *Getting Bitter or Getting Better*. He suggests that all of us would do well to recognize that:

♦ Negative feelings toward self are normal. This does not relieve us of responsibility for self-control. We can find better ways to express bad feelings without hurting self.
♦ We are human beings; human beings make mistakes. This is not because of destructive behavior. Rather, it is the basis for self-compassion and patience. Human beings can change and do change. Self forgiveness is an important avenue toward that goal.

- We do not have to feel worthy to forgive ourselves. That is why we deal with forgiveness rather than justice.
- Forgiving ourselves is important preparation for forgiving others. Choosing to love or hate ourselves influences how we see our environment and those who populate it. (p. 50)

My good friend, Rev. Dr. Bob, has worked with me for many years and is probably one of the most naturally receptive person I know, establishing relationships with people based on their souls, not on politics or ego. He has, it seems, been able to get beyond difference. Often, when I am in the middle of researching or writing on some topic, I will consult Bob for direction or advice. When I was focusing attention on forgiveness for this book, I asked Bob about his perspective. We had a great conversation, but he sensitized me to one key element with forgiveness – that it is often associated with being divine. In all of Bob's previous work as a minister and pastor, he found that forgiveness is thought to be fully operationalized in divine situations. The implication is that we mere mortals are incapable of forgiveness.

Now, I'm not so sure of this perspective. I know that forgiveness is not easy, but to position forgiveness as close to Godliness, suggests that most of us need not even try. It seems that if we are under the perception that this trait is so difficult to carry out, many will just give up the search.

I know, in my meager experiences and with those of my family and friends, that forgiveness is very difficult. Still, it is a trait that we must consider when thinking about difference. I believe that we mere mortals can operationalized forgiveness, but to do so must start with our feeling that we can. We must recognize that many among us have achieved a sense of forgiving those who have done wrong. One such story is that of Jackie Pflug.

Recently, I had chance to meet Jackie and to share a speaking engagement with her. Her story really starts back in 1987 when she was living and working in the Mediterranean with her husband. On a trip to Egypt with her husband, Jackie needed to head back to their home sooner than he. Halfway home, in the air, Jackie's flight was hijacked.

The terrorists had the plane land in Malta and demanded that it be refueled to fly to Libya. The Maltese government chose to not negotiate with the terrorists. To heighten the ante, the terrorists next announced that if their demands were not made, they would assassinate a passenger every 15 minutes. Still, the Maltese government held firm.

The terrorists then gathered all the passports, there were some 300 civilians on the flight. They called forward all the Israeli citizens, and then every 15 minutes they shot one in the head and pushed their bodies out the plane and on to the tarmac.

After all the Israeli's were assassinated, the terrorists called forward the American citizens. There were three, including Jackie Pflug.

As they sat together, praying and trying to console each other, the terrorists took the first American, an older man, placed a gun to his temple, and in front of Jackie and the other American, shot him in the head.

Fifteen minutes later, the next American man was pulled forward, knelt down, and again, in front of Jackie, shot in the head. She knew she was next to die.

As the minutes ticked away, Jackie told me she felt she had made peace and was ready to die. She was grabbed by the arm and put into a kneeling position. The gun was cocked and placed to her head. Next, she remembers feeling a strong thump on the side of her head, then a floating sensation, finally a rough, solid conclusion. In a surreal state, she wondered if heaven was this strange, solid place. Then she realized that she was not dead, but lying on the tarmac, underneath the hijacked plane.

For five hours, Jackie Pflug lay still on the tarmac, fearful that the terrorists would discover that she was still alive and finish the job. Soon, the airline was seized and in the battle many passengers were killed. It wasn't until the bodies were being hauled off to the morgue, that she was discovered alive.

After hearing Jackie's story, I was amazed with her perspective. Here was a vibrant woman, at the beginning of her career, newly married, whose dreams were put on hold. The bullet that ripped into her skull, though not lethal, penetrated into her temporal and parietal lobes causing many permanent changes. Her long rehabilitation and subsequent challenges pulled her marriage apart. She was told that she would never be able to go back to her occupational love – teaching. Her life was permanently altered.

Yet, she told me she had forgiven the terrorists. It had taken time, but she had arrived at a place where she felt these things had happened for a reason. She had forgiven.

In comparison to Jackie Pflug, most of our experiences of with pain and suffering seem to be minor. Imagine the intensity of being an innocent victim in someone's culture where you are slated to die; where you sit and watch others die, and then you are next. This kind of experience, when reflecting on my own situation with pain and suffering, is almost incomparable.

So this notion of forgiveness looms out there as a key spiritual trait that can get us beyond difference, and the pain, anger and hostility, associated with the wounding process. To really get beyond the emotions of difference, we must work at forgiveness.

Yet, forgiveness remains as the most difficult of traits in this exploration to achieve. How can we be more forgiving? Are there ways we can allow people the indiscretions the levy? This review is not designed to answer these questions, but to raise our consciousness around forgiving. We must enter forgiveness as key variable in getting beyond difference.

12

Reflections To Get Beyond Difference

12

Reflections To Get Beyond Difference

And so we come full circle. In many ways, to examine difference is to examine ourselves. We look out to differences and in the journey we must pass through our own spirits and hopefully find ourselves.

This exploration continues to be an interesting and illuminating one for me. My struggles in understanding how we relate to one another has been initially examined through the lens of human services. In this effort, I have attempted to understand behavior by considering the way our society deals with people who are at the fringe.

In my book, *Interdependence*, the trends and traditions of human services were outlined. It wasn't until after the book was published, however, that I truly focused on the internal/external struggle that precedes the formal treatment of people. Prior to this awareness, I felt that the problems we continue to face in supporting people at the fringe of society was more of a systems thing. I thought if we could only pass a law, or change a rule, things would get better. I did countless workshops and seminars on interdependence, empowerment, and advocacy. We need to change systems and people. Why couldn't people just think like me?

I'm not exactly sure when all this changed, but some way, some how, I began to reassess my thoughts and actions. Instead of looking outward, I began to look inward. Rather than seeing the problems from an external direction, I am now thinking more about my personal perspective. It seemed that the answers for change now fall more in the spiritual domain than in the systems domain.

Another new awareness I had was try as I might, there is no way I can change others. I finally realized that the only person I can change (and even that is an intense struggle) is me.

This is not to say that there is not an external systems agenda to consider. Indeed, there is, and any of us interested in change must be ready to go this route. There are also some key strategies and practical aspects of systems change that we must think about. Still, any external action is a reflection of current spirit and soul. Where we decide to go is dictated by where we are. We must understand our values, philosophy, and spirituality if we are to make any formidable change.

The internal/external struggle plays out in a number of ways. Given the constant tension between our individual drives vs. attention that must be given to the common good, we find ourselves in the state of flux. Indeed, on a larger scale, Robert Bellah and his associates (1991) focused on this when they stated:

> A successful life in American society depends on the ability to negotiate competently a series of requirements, primarily to show technical competence and secondarily to demonstrate the ability to deal with other people... Life in this paradigm is a competitive race to acquire the objective markers (college boards, admission to the right school, GPA, LSAT, advanced degree, entry to the right organizations, promotion to higher echelon positions) that give access to all the good things that make life worthwhile (attractiveness to desirable mate, purchase of an appropriate home, American Express Gold Card, vacations in Europe). But, what this form of life minimizes, if it does not neglect alto-

gether, is any larger moral meaning, any contribution to the common good, that might help it make sense... Beyond following the rules that tell us how to get ahead, we have trouble making moral sense of our immediate actions... We think what is required here is only a high level of competence, of expertise, of "professionalism," not the moral wisdom that should be the base of any good institution. And when things go wrong, we tend to blame individuals, we deny their lack of "ethics," but we don't question the morality of the institutions themselves. (pp. 42-43)

This notion of the struggle between individual achievement and the common good is clearly prevalent in all of our institutions. Time and again in my travels I find people from varying fields who testify to similar struggles that I find in the field of human services. Again, Bellah speaks to these trends from a sociological perspective:

There is a profound gap in our culture between technical reason, the knowledge with which we design computers or analyze the structure of DNA, and practical or moral reason, the ways we understand how we should live... But technical reason alone, as we have seen, is insufficient to manage our social difficulties or make sense of our lives. What we need to know is not simply how to build a powerful computer or how to redesign DNA but precisely and above all what to do with that knowledge. (pp. 46)

Our times are changing and we must appreciate an imbalance that may be occurring. A technical, mechanistic society without a moral, values base is a set up for distantiation and abuse.

Another purveyor of this struggle between individual drives and the common good is Amitai Etzioni, (1993). In 1990, he launched a movement toward "communitarianism." He states:

The communitarian movement – which is an environmental movement dedicated to the betterment of our moral, social and political environment – seeks to... bring about the changes in values, habits and public policies that will allow us to do for society what the environmental movement seeks to do for nature: to safeguard and enhance our future. (pp. 2-3)

Etizoni and his colleagues believe we must balance rights with the broader responsibilities we have to our communities. These responsibilities are to not only be good citizens, but to proactively safeguard the basic standards of society. It's a bold agenda.

Another reflection I have, as I close out this book, is that of incubation. I remember reading about creativity by the likes of Rollo May (1981), and most of those who examine this phenomena of creativity talk about incubation. May contends that when a problem or issue is presented to us, especially deeper more perplexing problems, they are not easily solved. It might be that we are not yet ready or that our existing paradigm keep giving us the same answer that continues to fall short. Then one day, perhaps long after the problem was introduced, an answer may seep into our consciousness. Some people refer to this as an "ah ha" experience. What causes this, and why it takes time is still not known. But we do know that incubation is an important part of the process. For me, with *Interdependence*, it took me a good six years before I clearly saw the essentialities of the inward road as opposed to the external route I was previously on.

Indeed, the "hatching" of the book, *Interdependence*, was also an incubation of the thoughts and notions of Goffman, Illich, Wolfensberger, and others. Their powerful ideas, most published in the 60s and 70s gave way to my perspectives on *Interdependence*.

And so for some, I hope *Beyond Difference* promotes an incubation about the notion of inclusion. As people hear, read, and think more about their spiritual side, I hope a "hatching" of new behaviors will occur. And as more people think and act on their consciousness with kindness, hospitality, generosity, compassion, and forgiveness, we will begin to see a critical mass toward change occur. In the spirited compilation, *Gifts of the Lotus*, this process is captured nicely with the following reflection:

> In each man is a spark able to kindle new fires of human progress, new light for the human spirit... When enough of these fires are burning, they create a new dawn of spiritual understanding; the flame of a great people is formed. (p. 155)

The Rev.. Dr. Bob recently gave me an interesting article by Frederick Buechner (1993) called "Journey Toward Wholeness." In it, Buechner examines the notion of wholeness and how difficult it is for people to get beyond brokenness, in a world riddled by famine and wars and political upheaval. He states:

> We are citizens of a nation that in all its history has perhaps never been so dramatically confronted as it is now by its brokenness... A nation whose city streets are littered by the bodies of the homeless and a fifth of whose children go to bed hungry at night if they are lucky enough to have beds, a nation that continues to spend billions on defense against the enemy without, when it becomes more apparent every day that all the real enemies are within – poverty, illiteracy, the despair that breeds crime and addiction. (p. 460)

Buechner's essay caught my attention because it parallels a point *Beyond Difference* attempts to make; that those of us caught up in the morass of a system, either because we are different, or are trying to address the problems of difference, the answers lie within, not without. We must understand that to charge forward to cry foul in addressing those that devalues us, (or those we love) is putting a bandage on a larger wound, rather than treating the wound. In understanding difference, the reasons for the wound are not the elements of the difference, but the inability of our spirits to embrace difference. We have so much inward work to do.

Fortunately, more current reality seems to be on this inward side. The President of the United States, Bill Clinton, campaigned to office, on a platform of inclusion. He challenged that we need all our citizens, that everyone should be at the table. Indeed, his deliberate actions are to be inclusive and welcoming to all the people of our society. He has strongly endorsed multi-culturalism.

Add to this, the passage of the Americans with Disabilities Act (ADA) in 1990 (PL 101-336). This landmark legislation is more than a civil rights bill for people with differences brought on by disabilities. Indeed the ADA rescripts society's perspectives on disability. As the act itself states:

> Some 43,000,000 Americans have one or more physical or mental disabilities, and this number is increasing as the population as a whole is growing older.

> Historically society has tended to isolate and segregate individuals with disabilities, and, despite some improvements, such forms of discrimination against individuals with disabilities continues to be serious and pervasive social problem...

> Individuals with disabilities continually encounter various forms of discrimination, including outright intentional exclusion, the discriminatory effects of architectural, transportation, and communication barriers. Overprotective rules and policies, failure to make modifications to existing facilities and practices, exclusionary qualifications, standards and criteria, segregation, and relegation to lesser services, programs, activities, benefits, jobs or other opportunities...

> Individuals with disabilities are a discreet and insular minority who have been faced with restrictions and limita-

tions, subjected to a history of purposeful unequal treatment and relegated to a position of political powerlessness in our society, based on characteristics that are beyond the control of such individuals and resulting from stereotypic assumptions not truly indicative of the individual ability of such individuals to participate in, and contribute to society. (p. 304)

These words of the ADA are powerful. They suggest that society has isolated and segregated, that it is discrimination, not individual differences that are the pervasive social problem and that disability is merely a characteristic, not some problem to be dealt with. These notions are at the core of this book. The problem is our inability, as individuals and as a society, to get beyond seeing and reacting to the difference of disability or any other type of difference for that matter.

In fact, the recently authorized Rehabilitation Act (PL 102-569) put forth by the United States Congress presents the same arguments. The Act states:

Disability is a natural part of human experience and in no way diminishes the right of individuals to live independently, enjoy self determination, make choices, contribute to society, pursue meaningful careers, and enjoy full inclusion and integration in the economic, political, social, cultural and educational mainstream of American Society.

For those interested in disability as a type of difference, this statement is a landmark. It asserts that disability is not some aberration, but a natural part of the human experience. For time in memorial, people with disabilities were treated as if they are the problem, that they need to be fixed, and until they change, must be segregated into a world that could "take care of them." The Rehabilitation Act says loud and clear that the medical expert approach is not the way to address disability. We need to see people with disabilities from the light of their capacities. We must be able to get beyond difference.

Another concluding point is to reflect on the language we use to describe people and events. The effects of labeling people was examined in the text of this work. Without question labels given to people, no matter how noble their intent, tend to offset, stereotype and stigmatize people. To get beyond difference is to become sensitive to the terms used to describe difference. This is easier said than done. In fact, to a certain extent, to drop our labels is a type of paradox. The current approach is to use labels to understand difference, yet when we use these labels they tend to polarize. If we drop labels, how do we come to describe people's uniqueness? In fact, do we have to describe people's uniqueness at all?

These questions are not easily answered. We are so conditioned to talk about people through their descriptive labels, that we seemingly know no other way. They are "African American men," or "disabled person," or "tall woman." Whatever, these descriptors have become common place in our life, language, actions, and style. Since we don't acknowledge their potentially wounding effect, we don't bat an eye when we use them.

We must awaken to the power of language. The words we use have deep impact on the people we relate with and to a society in general. We must find a way to be conscious and consistent with the words we use. This consciousness should emanate from the traits of kindness, hospitality, generosity, compassion and forgiveness — especially if we are working to get beyond difference.

Further, we need to create a consistent blend between the words we use and the actions we show. That is, if we speak to the notion of inclusion, as the ADA and Rehabilitation Act suggest, then we must understand the word and embrace its connotation. Inclusion is a strong word, with a clear value attached to it. Inclusion implies that all are welcomed into the discourse. It also suggests that people do not have to be fixed or change to participate. Rather, people should be included as they are. It allows for a flexibility and a fluidity of acceptance for culture, physical, or cognitive difficulties. It has the values base of kindness and hospitality oozing from it.

I first became sensitive to the notion of inclusion after reading a thoughtful interview of the playwright August Wilson by Bill Moyers done in 1987. Wilson, a native of Pittsburgh and Pulitzer Prize winning author, has been outspoken critic in race relations. In the interview, Moyers asked Wilson how he felt the cause of integration was fairing in America. Crisp and to the point, Wilson said, "I don't believe in integration." An obviously stunned Moyers pressed on and Wilson continued to describe how integration is about accepting another person's standards. Rather than to be accepted for his blackness, Wilson contended that integration pushed him to fit into a white culture. He felt that his blackness and the reality of his own culture was (and is) not acknowledged in the goal of integration.

If you examine the word *inclusion*, or the root word *include* in a dictionary, you find that it means being a part of or member of a group or association. Even more focused are the words listed as synonyms to the word include. They are comprise, comprehend, embrace, and involve. These works all speak to a bonding or melding of person and spirit into the fold. Quite simply, the word inclusion implies some action.

As we reflect on the word *inclusion*, it also calls us to examine our own actions as well. Before we can say to the community, "you need to be inclusive of people who are different," we must first answer this question ourselves. How inclusive are we in our own lives? How inclusive are the networks, groups, and associations of which we are members? How welcoming of diversity are the very patterns that we keep?

My own reflections on these matters have been illuminating. When I think of most of the worlds I keep, they are not as inclusive as I would like them to be. Our agency, UCP of Pittsburgh, for all intents and purposes, has been an exclusive domain for people with disabilities. Until we started our conscious effort to be an inclusive community center, we stood as some separate place where people with disabilities should go to be changed by special programs. Other groups that I relate to, my church, the little league association, our school's PTG, and others, are relatively insular and narrow in membership. Granted, these groups may have a parochial agenda, but even with this, I would think that people with some observable difference could be a part. Where are they? Why aren't they in my circles?

Such reflection is causing me to not only center myself around issues such as inclusion, but act on them as well. Every day, in many ways, I have opportunity to ask about, or more importantly, model the actions of inclusion. I am now trying to live the solution rather than to advocate for it.

It's interesting though, the pitfalls I find in this process. And they are found not just with others, but within me as well. A couple of internal struggles revolve around convenience, speed, and consciousness.

The first of these is consciousness. As was mentioned earlier in this work, any actions of personal change require an acknowledgment to act at all. Many times, I breeze about my personal life without keeping the action of inclusion as a part of it. I simply don't have it in my consciousness. When I do however, inclusion is still a struggle. I find that to take the time to include people requires not only time, but it also might take me out of my way. Even simple inconveniences of driving an extra mile to pick someone up or drop a person off offers me an excuse not to include. I tell myself that it pulls me too much out of my way. Or, I use the excuse of how long it might take to include people and that I just don't have the time. I keep promising myself that come tomorrow I will make more time, and then I never do.

These internal battles, I have learned, are ones that other people I know and respect share, and struggle with. Equally challenging, is trying to bring the actions of inclusion to rest with the organizations I am part of. For example, one would think that the actions of inclusion, especially as we have used them in this book, would be "easy" to pull off with my organization, UCP of Pittsburgh. Yet, years of crust and hardening related to the traditional ways we have served people with disabilities have created incredible anchors. At every turn, it seems there is another reason, seemingly justifiable, that creates a road block in a more pure realization of inclusion. Either we don't have enough support people, or funds, or the funding source won't allow it, or the rationalization that inclusion just can't happen for some people. Probably the stronger perversion is the notion that people with significant difference just don't want to be included.

Now, I don't know about you, but I can recall times that I was not included and they were never pleasant experiences. I do know that often, after feeling the pangs of exclusion, I would announce that I didn't want to be a part of the group anyway. It was sort of a defense to be able to rationalize the hurt of exclusion.

To a large extent, these organizational struggles can also be tied to the notions of convenience and speed. Since organizations are a collection of people toward a common cause, the values, personality and character of these organizations become a mirror of its members. If members, such as myself, can find convenience, speed, or consciousness as excuses to not be more inclusive in my own life then so too, can others at our agency. Just like people, our organization is moving at a certain pace, looking for efficient and convenient ways to carry out our business. All of this leads to a collective unconsciousness to the notions of inclusion.

Many of us who work for UCP have thought long and hard about this organizational struggle. As we analyze our culture and look to change, one point of focus revolves around the values base of our organizational. Like many human service agencies that specialize in disability issues, our values base is a simple notion that all people, regardless of situation or circumstance are entitled to dignity, respect and a chance to participate. Over the past 10 years, however, we have not paid real attention to these values. The results have been a drifting from some of these beliefs and some clear rationalizations when we have acknowledged the drifting.

The bottom line is basic. If the goal of our individual or organizational efforts is to include, then we should just do it. Either people with difference are included into the groups and associations of community or they are not. In many ways, our specialities, jargon, and professionalism have gotten in our way.

GETTING BEYOND DIFFERENCE

Getting beyond difference takes an awareness, a consciousness and some tangible actions. Seeing people from a focus of kindness and hospitality, for many of us, must be relearned. In the previous sections, we have examined difference and the traits that are critical to growing beyond our propensity to see difference. Now we turn our attention to some tangible actions – things that might help us keep

Work of the eye is done, now go and do heart work.
Rilke

our consciousness up and spirit focused. Know that these ideas are not meant to be a self help menu. Indeed, without the basics of the aforementioned traits in place, any items reviewed here will be hollow. But, with the right frame of consciousness these items might be instructive. Most of these notions are ones I have observed, heard others speak of, or try to do myself.

READ

To get beyond difference implies a willingness to learn, grow and open to diversity. A great precursor to this type of growth can be found through reading. For every item explored throughout this book there are fantastic resources available to push you further. Some of these resources are listed in this book's Reference section, others are just a library or bookstore away.

It is really interesting to me, how little people read these days. Our society has become so visual/mass media oriented that most people have become habituated to television and movie orientation to information. People just find it easier, faster or more convenient to get news, views, stories, and directions from the screen, tapes, or radio. The notion of curling up with a good book seems not only ancient to some people, but in some circles, cause for jokes. An interesting testimony to how far we are drifting from reading, happened to me a few months ago while off on a trip.

I was in a hotel in Chicago and decided to get a sandwich and beer in the hotel sports bar. Since I never go anywhere without some reading material, I carried a book to the bar. Sitting off in the corner, I got caught up in my book and lost track of time. Although I wasn't paying much attention, I soon realized that the bartenders were playing a sort of trivia game with the customers, asking questions and rewarding the right answers with a drink.

After a few questions had passed, the bartender said, "I've got a good one. We'll give a free drink to the first customer who can show us a library card." I noticed that a dull silence seemed to fall over the bar and no one had a library card. When it was clear no one was coming forward, I pulled out my trusty Carnegie Library card, rushed up to the bar, then collecting my beer, sat back to ponder the magnitude of this experience.

There were at least 100 people in this bar, most well dressed, obviously professional people. The hotel was a Marriott, certainly not a "Rod's Roadside Motel." I'm sure most of the guests were successful business people, fairly well educated. Still, not one person had a library card. Now, maybe most people don't travel with their library cards, perhaps to keep them safe and secure from hotel thieves. Or, maybe most of the guests had lent their library cards out. Or maybe, just maybe, most of these particular guests didn't have a library card.

I don't know about you, but I remember when I first got my library card. I was just a tot at my dad's side when he signed me up. Perhaps it was the way my dad handled it, but I remember it as an incredibly important day and an experience that etched into my memory. As we walked down those quiet aisles, the book shelves seemed like mountains. In many regards, it was like being in church, reverent, dignified, and important.

To this day, I am a library affectionado. I seek them out and feel safe in their bosom. When I travel, I try to make a point to visit the local public library. Indeed, you can tell the character of a town or city, by its library. I particularly like college and university libraries.

A final point about libraries, was the feeling I had recently when I enrolled my own children at the Carnegie Library of Pittsburgh. How proud they were to have their own card and now we make a regular trek to the library every two weeks. I want my children to feel home there, to revel in the smell and sounds, to appreciate the majesty of books and reading. We must, as Crosby, Stills and Nash contended, teach our children well.

Often, people who know my passion for reading seem amazed at how I can find time. They often lament that they are just too busy, can't fit any more into their day. These kind of responses are curious to me. Please know that my schedule is just as busy as the next person. I manage a major human service agency with a 4 million dollar budget, I'm involved in more of my fair share of human services committees, boards, and coalitions. My work week, like many of yours, averages 50 to 60 hours. On top of all this is my traveling and speaking schedule.

Over the past five years, I have averaged 20 major presentations each year, most out of town requiring at least one overnight. Then, add to this my community and civic work — president of my children's school's PTG, involved with our church and helping to coach two little league teams, as well. Finally, though not at all last on the list, is my family. With three children under 11 years of age, I have important daddy duties which I take very seriously. Still, I find time to read. I am convinced that we all have more time in our busy schedules than we acknowledge. We just need to seize it.

One rule of thumb I like to keep is to always try to read things that are recommended by people I respect. I can't remember a time that I was let down by someone's suggestion. I also try to stay exposed to a broad range of writings. Not only between fiction/non fiction, but writings by authors that come from other fields or perspectives.

Indeed, if we expect reading to help us grow we must be ready to expand to writings that might challenge our perspectives. When we do this we are called to defend our beliefs, within the scope of the other's argument. This can't help but keep us sharp.

Another thought about reading comes with an intimacy of books. To me, a book is an interactive vessel, one that involves interchange. Often, when I get strong feelings about a passage I might read, I try to make a point to underscore or to write my comments in the margins of the page. This type of interaction tends to the immediacy of reading. When we do this, it causes us to take a stand, focus our thoughts. It also makes your books highly personal. They truly become yours when you mark them up, and allow you a point of history and presence when you come back to them later.

My "book club" friends and I are always fascinated by each other's markings. When I share books with the Rev. Dr. Bob, the things he has marked always help me better understand his character and passions. These markings are interesting road maps to better knowing your friends.

So read, explore, examine, research, dig, learn how to find things, but by all means read. It is an essential element to keeping our consciousness high. Reading, as they say, is fundamental to growth.

REFLECTION

To read is but a start point to the process of growth. One must also reflect, and reflection is a multi-phased phenomena. Of course, the first step to reflection is found with an initial "hit" of the passage read. Unless, we push ourselves to be with the passage, these "hits" might just pass us by. For me, to read an important passage aloud really helps drive it home. At times, this activity can seem odd. Especially, when you are on a plane or sitting by a pool. That is why my preference is to read a passage aloud to someone else and get their thoughts. Although I try to do this with people I know, from time to time I have done it with strangers. You need To appreciate that although this is a risk (some folks might think you a bit odd) it is incredible the conversations you will inspire. I've met some fascinating people by reading to them.

Of course, the best experience of reflection is found when a group of people read the same thing and then come together to discuss it. This format is one used in many colleges, though for most students, the books/articles are not theirs to choose. The selections are from the faculty and the whole process becomes an "assignment" designed to get a grade. Maybe this initial forced method of academic reflection is one of the reasons many of us shy away from this type of exercise once we finish school. It's sort of a conditioned reflex bore from an initially bad experience; and so we steer clear. Still, to read something together and then discuss its impact is a method bound to promote reflection. Book clubs or reading partners are excellent vehicles to reflection.

Another form of reflection to passages read, is to write a response or reaction. This exercise can be taxing because it forces us to commit to paper our feelings and reactions. There is a big difference between the spoken reflection and the written reflection. The spoken reflection can evaporate after it has been said — the written word lives on. Unless destroyed, it becomes a permanent record. Know, however, that it is often difficult to push beyond our written comments. They seemingly live with us.

A good example of the power, and to a certain extent, anchor of the written word is found in the analysis conducted on political or judicial appointments. Whenever a new political appointment is made to the Supreme Court, for example, the Senate Judiciary Committee, as well as lobbyists, pro and con, and reporters too, scurry to find out who the candidate really is through their previously written opinions. To a lesser extent, many of us can relate to the power of this phenomena when we find a box of our old college papers while cleaning the attic. This recently happened to me and I sat in a dusty, ill lit cubby hole, pouring over paper after paper muttering, "I can't believe I wrote this."

Still, there is no exercise of reflection more focused than writing it down. Many people keep a daily journal of their life reflections in a diary and this effort helps them get a handle on feelings. Reflective writings, once we get over the fears of revealing our thoughts, can be one of the most clarifying experiences a person can have.

OBSERVATION

Another way to keep conscious and to learn about the traits that can help us get beyond difference, is to watch out for them. I am constantly scanning my environment for examples of kindness, hospitality, generosity, compassion, and forgiveness. Most often, I look for these activities in everyday experiences. When I find them, I try to analyze their flow, pick apart the elements that define them — such as the factors that make my Aunt Nat generous, or my Aunt Dolly hospitable. I try to cull out the things that are structural parts to their acts of generosity and hospitality.

Further removed, I also try to find the salient features of acts that I observe between strangers, like the observations I have made in airports or acts of kindness found at gatherings. Although you may not know the players, these actions can be equally instructive.

Other important venues of observation, are restaurants. Since meals play such an important role in ceremonies and celebrations, restaurants become a prime spot to ferret out acts of hospitality, compassion, or kindness. Watching people's affect as they cement this ceremony can offer strong lessons. An even stronger lesson can be learned by paying attention to toasts people make. In fact, it seems that the time honored tradition of toast making is dying out. In my family, for example, the torch has passed to me to be the official toast maker. When I prod others to speak up, they defer pointing out that I'm the outspoken "Condeluci".

Still, another setting to observe spiritual acts, especially the notion of compassion, is at funeral homes. To see how people reach out with body and words to console the bereaved offers great opportunity to reflect and learn. One strong teacher for me in these settings in my sister, Jan. As the eldest in our family, Jan is a study in warmth and compassion at family wakes. She has a strong, but silent presence and just standing there holding hands with the family speaks volumes in compassion.

A final dimension of observation can be found with entertainment or media. A movie or a play can tell you so much about compassion or forgiveness. Forget the fact that its a story or script and focus on the details of how the character manifests any of the traits we have discussed. To this extent, all life becomes a classroom to understanding our spirits.

MODEL

As simple as it may sound, or as stilted as it may seem, probably the best way to push the development of any of these traits is to practice them. Like most physical endeavors, we can only get better at something if we practice it. So is this true for our spirits, as well as our bodies. To this extent, actually reminding yourself to be kind or hospitable, to practice a handshake that projects warmth, to go out of your way to compliment someone, are all ways that we can get better at the spiritual domain.

To this end, it is amazing to me that many of us in human services promote a notion of inclusion for the people we support, yet do not actually do it ourselves. My friend, Mark Johnson, asks pointedly in his talks, "How many people working for disability rights live in an accessible home?" Or similarly, "How many people working for state welfare systems have close friends who use welfare." The point is that we have to practice what we preach. How can we ask people in the community to do that which we have not done ourselves? Simple, yet powerful reality.

And so is true for the spiritual domain. If the thesis in this book makes any sense to you in helping us get beyond difference, then to not attempt to practice these spiritual traits is to be hypocritical. This is also why practice and modeling are such an important part of honing or developing the spiritual skills necessary to get beyond difference. So don't miss a chance to work on your style and approach in being as kind, generous, hospitable, compassionate, and forgiving as possible. Not only will your efforts help you further develop your skills, but you will be amazed at the rewards that will follow; the doors that will open and the impact that will occur.

COMPLIMENT AND ACKNOWLEDGE

Psychologists know that one way to harden a behavior is to reinforce its action through reward so that actions can be "modified." One powerful type of reward, is a compliment or kind word. Given this reality, a strong way to promote the behaviors that will help us get beyond difference is to recognize, and then acknowledge, positive spiritual behavior through a compliment.

The next time you witness an act of kindness, or hospitality or any of the others, tell the person you respect their actions. Let them know that the world is that much better because of them; that they are making a difference in creating a better community.

Often, in the workshops I do, I'll ask those in attendance to think of the kindest person they know. (In fact, that challenge was made in the earlier section on kindness.) After people have a chance to identify that kindest person they know, I ask them to do one more thing — to let that person know they thought of them in this way the next time they see them.

We can't let these positive moments pass. When people you know (or even don't know) go out of their way for another, they should be rewarded; and all it takes is the consciousness to do it.

The management expert, Tom Peters, knows this power well. In his writings, he urges managers to wonder around their organizations and catch people doing things right; and then let them know. This immediate attention to positive behavior is a powerful management tool. So too, can we enhance spiritual growth by acknowledging and complementing the everyday acts of generosity.

My colleague, Mary Lou Busby, is a master at this. She has a deep spirit and is a wonderful manager. Not only does she compliment people immediately, she also captures it in a hand written note to the person and copies me in the process. This way, the people who work with her know that I know they are doing a great job.

TEACH

All of us, to a greater or lesser degree, play some formalized role as a teacher. It might be with our children, or as a coach, or as a friend, or in actual teaching positions. Whatever and whenever, we should not miss the opportunity to teach others about the benefits of the traits we are examining in this book.

I know that in my most important role of a teacher – with my children, I can think of no more critical or fundamental lesson to share with Dante, Gianna, and Santino, than that of kindness. This seems especially true in a world that is becoming increasingly violent. In these lessons, Liz and I try to be as rewarding and acknowledging of their kind acts as we are of a report card full of A's.

Now, this might seem elementary, but I'm not so sure how many people really learn the lessons of basic social relations with others that leads to the actions we are exploring here. I remember talking with my son, Dante, actually teaching him how to shake hands and greet a guest. He needed to learn how to offer a firm grip, to look directly at the person and offer them something to make them feel at home. Often, we seem to take these basic things for granted, as if people will naturally develop them. One look around, however, at the many people who are socially uncomfortable, and to a certain extent, inept, should tell us that many of these actions need to be taught. I still find myself struggling to learn the nuances of social graces.

I remember another example, where teaching these spiritual traits played a key role. It was with my son's little league team I helped coach last year. As I observed the other coaches focusing on teaching the skills of baseball, I felt it equally important that we teach the players the elements of teamwork, good sportsmanship, cooperation, and hospitality. While the other coaches worked on batting and throwing, I was working on kindness and generosity. These elements made for not only a successful team on the field, but a solid team in the dugout, and off the field, as well.

We must always be alert to the opportunities we have to not only be good models, the most powerful form of teaching, but to be instructors of actions, as well. In my work role, I do my best to weave lessons of these spiritual traits into the actions of supervision. We talk often of how we must keep our organization hospitable, responsive, and generous. To this point, I read an excellent book by James Autry (1991) titled, *Love and Profit*. Autry, the CEO of a large publishing firm, is convinced that the work place, in many regards, is complementing, or in some cases, replacing the family. He argues that with the transiency of the average worker and reduction of family size in general, the family has lost its place in many people's lives. Still, the important spiritual dimensions, usually filled by families, are needed by us all. His suggestion is that the workplace needs to serve this role and function more like a family.

TOUCH

One of the most basic needs of human beings is that of touch. When we reach out to people in a physical way, it leaves a powerful message. Indeed, from the famous Michelangelo painting in the Sistine Chapel of the hands extending to touch, the poignant moment in the movie, *ET* when Elliott and ET embrace, the notion of touch is symbolic of all the traits we have explored in this work.

Ironically, however, in our current day and age, the notion of touch must be balanced. For as warm of a concept as it is, touch has also been associated with the darker side of humanity, through acts of assault, violence, abuse, and molestation. Time and again, we see or read devastating stories where the notion of touch has not been reciprocal and violations have been levied. Probably most outrageous are the touching violations when one party has been misled, lured, or confused into compliance.

These types of experiences or publicly announced actions have had a serious affect on how our culture and institutions now interpret touch. In a sad sort of way, the rule of thumb today is to not touch another, steer clear, or stay aloof. Many formal human service organizations have adopted anti touch policies between employees and "clients" It's sort of a "better safe than sorry" approach to human services. Add to this, the current social interpretations of touching and the issue gets further clouded. A man touching a woman who is not his wife can be interpreted as a sexual advance. Even more, men who touch other men are almost always looked upon as possible acts of homosexuality.

As I write these words, I am called to an experience I had in Edmonton, Alberta, while at a conference that examined the spiritual side of rehabilitation work. At the end of the conference, my friend, Patrick, was summarizing and thanking participants. For each of us who presented, he had a small gift of appreciation. Now, I had only recently met Pat, first by phone in setting up the conference and then face to face when he picked me up at the airport. Still I felt a real bond of common interest and actions for change. After giving me the gift, we hugged warmly in front of the audience – not something uncommon for me. Later, that night at dinner, Patrick's wife said she bumped into one of the conference participants who quickly reported to her that we had hugged. The person had insinuated something more from the hug. It is a shame that the simple action of touching has grown to be feared or misinterpreted.

And so I reject these notions. Touching is vital to the human experience and I believe we are lesser when we limit it. I am a toucher and although I respect other people's space, I usually follow my basic instinct to touch. Usually, my hugs are warmly reciprocated.

It seems to me that to actualize kindness, hospitality, generosity, compassion, and forgiveness without touch dilutes the process. This doesn't mean we abuse the notion of touch. Rather, touching becomes a powerful vehicle when we act spiritually.

Celebrate

Often when I think about spirituality, I think about celebration at the same time. Maybe this relates to my association of celebrations as being tied to spiritual themes. We celebrate Christmas, (the spirit of the born savior); or July 4th, (the spirit of independence); or birthdays, (the spirit of life); or Thanksgiving, (the spirit of thanks). For me, these, and other holidays, bring back warm feelings of family gatherings, food, song, dance, and stories. They also bring to mind smiles, laughter, and happiness.

Celebrations, to me, are a melting of the traits we have discussed. Like a gestalt, they fuse together to create a dynamic and impactful embodiment of the spirit. These celebrations call forth laughter and smiles, a reawakening of the common humanity among us.

Recently, at a family Labor Day gathering on "Condeluci Hill," as the party was winding down, we found ourselves thinking back to past celebrations. My Aunt Betty, whose vivid mind serves as our family historian, was recounting these moments. What suddenly hit me, as she spoke, was the spiritual presence of our family members who have passed before.

In my mind, I saw again Uncle Jim, Aunt Jeannette, Uncle Pete, and the many others who, though gone from this earth, are still a part of our family celebrations. Thinking about them, and the fun or humorous stories woven by Aunt Betty, pushed me to intensify the need for the "Beyond Difference Traits" in my own life. This celebration was more than the moment but caused reflection both of the past and toward the future.

Recently, I asked some friends what emotions were conjured up when thinking about the five traits of this book. The question was simple — what emotion, happy or sad, goes with the trait? Although not scientific (in fact while telling these results to a scientific friend of mine, he inquired as to the statistical significance of the responses) let me assure you here, Chi Square aside, these responses are anecdotal, but interesting none the less. They were:

> kindness — happy
> hospitality — happy
> generosity — happy
> compassion — sad
> forgiveness — sad

What are your thoughts here?

As it relates to celebration, it seems that to celebrate kindness, hospitality, and generosity with smiles, laughter, and song should be easy. But can we celebrate compassion and forgiveness, the traits most people I talked to associated with sadness? My friend, Reverend Doctor Bob, says, "Yes!" In fact, he feels that, both compassion and forgiveness, because they push us a little harder, are cause indeed, for celebration. He says that being able to act upon suffering ignites our common humanity and anything that does this is celebratory. And, forgiveness, arguably the most challenging of the traits to truly realize, once achieved, should be pause to serve the fatted calf.

And so, celebrate these traits and be sure to reflect upon your celebration. Further, bring others into your celebration and everyone benefits. Life is too short to do otherwise.

Conclusion

*Be kind. Remember, everyone you
meet is fighting a hard battle.*
                                    T. H. Thompson

Conclusion

All things, more or less, have a natural cycle. They start out with much hope and, at times, fanfare. This newness gives way to a middle period where things get done, a settling in occurs, and the actions play out. Then finally, a concluding point comes where the notion ends. Sometimes, these conclusions are abrupt, leaving us to want more. At other times, the conclusions drag on, well beyond their impact. The ideal, however, is when conclusion occurs at just the right time — one that leaves those around satisfied. Such, I hope, is the case with this book.

It was designed as an effort to examine difference and then offer inward reflections for ways to get beyond the throes of difference. Taking the adage that the only person we can truly change is ourselves, this work was more of process for internal change. Although it poses some organizational questions, it is etched more from the premise that to embrace difference we must not only understand our spiritual side, but to let it come out.

Of all the spiritual notions that could have been considered, I chose the traits of kindness, hospitality, generosity, compassion, and forgiveness. I readily admitted the limitations of these variables and some readers might be inclined to add others. Indeed, my friend, Janet Williams, in learning of the five traits, wondered why "hope" wasn't included. As a specialist in family issues, she told me how important hope is to parents and children who might experience significant difference. She makes a good point. Hope is an important variable. Again, I state loud and clear, the spiritual issues explored in this work do not purport to be the best or the only ones. (Hey, Janet, maybe this is our chance to write together about hope.) Still, the traits covered are ones that can be helpful.

Another goal of this work was to use a style that is informal, anecdotal, and friendly. Although I tried to anchor, document, and focus points to solid, academic roots, I feel strongly that too much of the literature on the topic of difference is overly academic and hard to follow. Further, since the mainstay of this text looked at spiritual matters, I feel it is essential to keep things readable. In this effort, however, I hope my more academic friends do not shy away. We must balance our work, and the influences of our effort must include spiritual grist as well as technical elements. This book, I hope, offers basics on both points.

As I conclude this work, I would be remiss not to, again, thank the many people who helped me etch this thesis. From folks who attended talks I have given, to those who I have had discussions with more depth. From my hometown of Pittsburgh, to San Diego, Tampa, Little Rock, Richmond, Rochester, Edmonton, and all those other cities, large and small in between. From people I know well and work with daily, to those that I met fleetingly. It was these people who focused, changed, edited, enhanced, or expanded the ideas that I have written about here. To all of you, I say, "Thanks." Many I have acknowledged in the afterword section.

And so, the time comes to put this book to bed. It has been two years now, since I began writing it, stealing time here and there, most often using airplane, airport, or hotel time to write. In fact, it is poetic that as I pen these words I sit on a moaning Northwest jet, somewhere over the great lakes. But the sky is bright and the clouds are magical and I feel happy to be going home. Also happy to be finishing this up. It has been a labor of love and clarification.

Know too, that since I am sure to be on more planes and caught in future airports there are other things to write. Just looming down the road is a planned book I am calling, *Strategies for Change*. This work will be the natural next step from *Beyond Difference* – a book that explores the external actions of change. If you have enjoyed *Beyond Difference* and *Interdependence*, *Strategies for Change* may be of interest to you, although I can't promise when it will be ready.

So for now, I better close. In some ways, I feel like I'm finishing a letter to a friend. Over the months it seems we have kicked around some important things. In fact, you can't find more important notions than kindness, hospitality, generosity, compassion, and forgiveness. So thanks for joining me on this journey. I feel like I have a better grip on the steering wheel and a clearer direction from the map. I look forward to the chance of talking with you down the road.

P.S. Don't forget to write back!

Afterword

*I am not one of those who think
that people are never in the wrong.
They have been so, frequently and
outrageously. But I do say that in all
disputes between them and their
rulers, the presumption is, at least
upon a par, in favor of the people.*

E. Burke

Afterword

A couple of years ago, I had the opportunity to attend a retreat at the Highlander Center in New Market, Tennessee. Although the gathering was specific to diversity issues, I was excited about spending time at the Highlander. For those who may not know, The Highlander Center is a school that focuses on social change. In its history, the union movement, civil rights movement, and ecological movement, have all had roots there. People like Rosa Parks, Martin Luther King, and Eleanor Roosevelt all spent time at the Center. The spirit of the Highlander is that people know their problems best and, given the opportunity, they know the solutions as well. Folks at the Center contend that the best expert is the person who is at the core of the problem or situation. In this perspective, we are all, indeed, experts.

I was changed at the Highlander Center by this perspective-changed in that I was given the power, along with the others in my group, to explore and solve our struggles. I was renewed to the potential we all have and how important and helpful our opinions can be. Like many other people, I had been lured into the false perspective that the expert or specialist, in whatever field, is essential to solving problems. The Highlander experience taught me differently.

In some ways, this experience also set me on the course of this book. I was inspired to not only look inward, but to examine the instincts and perspectives of people around me. As the topic of this book is truly about the human spirit, all of us could serve as ones to explore and clarify these traits. Although opinions of experts can be interesting and, at times, helpful, the perspectives of everyday people are real.

To this end, *Beyond Difference* has been sharpened and detailed by the ideas and experiences of many people. Although assemblage and interpretation of these vignettes are my own, I am remiss to not further acknowledge their input and contribution to this book.

So what follows is a listing of many of my friends or associates who have offered ideas, thoughts, or recommendations to the concepts in this work. These folks are listed by name and city and I have had direct conversations on these themes with them all. They are good people, all, and are proof that people do indeed know their own reality. All we have to do is simply listen!

Jack and Maryjo Allen	Carnegie, PA
Joe Aniello	Miami, FL
Jeff Armstrong	Boulder, CO
Kathy Armstrong	Boulder, CO
Joe Ashley	Richmond, VA
Judy Barricella	Pittsburgh, PA
Beth Beale	Portland, ME
Bob Beale	Portsmouth, ME
Dave Benjamin	Salsbury, MD
Allen Bergman	Washington, DC
JB Black	Tallahasse, FL
Jim Borin	Detroit, MI
Trevor Boyle	Belfast, Ireland
Bob Braden	Alexandria, VA
Fr. John Brennan	Kennedy, PA
Concetta Buiyak	McKees Rocks, PA
Lorraine Camenzoli	San Diego, CA
Jack and Marie Catanzarite	Hopewell, PA
Elmer Cerano	Detroit, MI
Bill Chrisner	Pittsburgh, PA
Dan Cohen	Pittsburgh, PA
Dave Condeluci	Crafton, PA
Frank Condeluci	McKees Rocks, PA
Gloria Condeluci	McKees Rocks, PA
Jane Condeluci	McKees Rocks, PA
Sarah Condeluci	McKees Rocks, PA

Sinbad Condeluci	McKees Rocks, PA
Tony and Rita Condeluci	McKees Rocks, PA
Will Condeluci	McKees Rocks, PA
Steve Cosgrove	Auburn, AL
Jim Costello	Tallahasse, FL
Jim Cunningham	Pittsburgh, PA
Jo Ann Davis Zucik	Ham, Ontario
Jim De Jong	Columbia, MO
Eva DisCasmirro	Vancouver, WA
Karen Engro	Pittsburgh, PA
Bill English	Tallahasse, FL
Fred Enck	Leesberg, FL
Dolly Fallon	Alexandria, VA
Mus Fallon	Alexandria, VA
Kevin and Eileen Finnigan	Kennedy Township, PA
Rick Forkosh	St. Louis, MO
John Freeland	Pamona, CA
Suzanne Gabel	Des Moines, IA
Steve Gieber	Sitluna, KS
Ralph and Sandy Gordon	Kennedy Township, PA
Sharon Gretz	Cheswick, PA
Sue Gunn	Columbia, MO
Greg Gwisdalla	Waterford, MI
Mark Hassemer	Columbia, MO
Linda Hinton	Des Moines, IA
Patrick Hirshe	Edmonton, Alberta
Bob Hogan	Las Vegas, NV
Rev. Al Hoogewind	Grand Rapids, MI
Kenny Hosak	Denver, CO
Brad Howell	Baltimore, MD
Rich Hubert	Turtle Creek, PA
Suzy Hutchinson	Stuart, FL
Jody Jackson	Durham, NC
Joe Johnson	Fischerville, VA
Mark Johnson	Atlanta, GA

Tom Kearney	Pittsburgh, PA
Dan Keating	Philadelphia, PA
Don and Lisa Kelley	Kennedy Township, PA
John Kemp	Washington, DC
Brian Klafane	Rochester, NY
Jeff Kreutzer	Richmond, VA
Dennis Lauria	McKees Rocks, PA
Natalie Lauria	McKees Rocks, PA
Betsy Lynem	Rochester, NY
Danese Malkamus	San Diego, CA
PJ Manuelian	Oklahoma City, OK
Rob Matevish	Fort Lauderdale, FL
Ed Mathews	New York
Bill McDowell	Pittsburgh, PA
Rev. Dr. Bob Miller	Wilmerding, PA
Michael Morris	Washington, DC
Don Morray	Lincoln, NE
Joe Morrone	Boston, MA
Thomas Neuville	Denver, CO
Bob Nelkin	Pittsburgh, PA
J. Dennis O'Conner	Pittsburgh, PA
Cheryl Palmer	Farmington Hills, MI
Phil Pappas	Piitsburgh, PA
Jim and Sandy Pastin	Kennedy Township, PA
John and Arlene Pastin	Orlando, FL
Jackie Pflug	Minneapolis, MI
Diana Ploof	Pittsburgh, PA
Ian Pumpian	San Diego, CA
Ray Remple	St. Catharines, Ontario
Peter Rumney	Toronto, CA
Fr. Regis Ryan	McKees Rock, PA
Janet Samuelson	Manassas, VA
Bill Sandonato	Clearwater, FL
Frank Savastano	Fort Lauderdale, FL
Vince and Cathy Sangricco	McKees Rocks, PA

Jim and Peggie Schweitzer	Kennedy Township, PA
Brad Sewick	Detroit, MI
Jordan Sher	San Diego, CA
Steve Sheridan	Philadelphia, PA
Christine Rafferty Shut	Cavroy, IN
Bob Spencer	Wilmington, DE
Jake Spisak	McKees Rocks, PA
Lucy Spruill	Piitsburgh, PA
Paul Stabile	Rapid City, SD
Gail Steiger	Rapid City, SD
Betty Straccia	McKees Rocks, PA
Pete Swales	Springville, NY
Bud Thoune	Seattle, WA
Jeff Tiesen	St. Catharines, Ontario
Jan Uhler	McKees Rocks, PA
Joe Uhler	McKees Rocks, PA
Susan Urofsky	Richmond, VA
Bob Walsh	Rochester, NY
David Weatherow	Winnipeg, Manitoba
Harry White	Pittsburgh, PA
Janet Williams	Kansas City, KS
Pat Yeager	San Diego, CA
Bruce Zewe	Freehold, NJ

References and Related Readings

References and Related Readings

American Heritage Dictionary - 3rd Edition. (1992). New York: Houghton Mifflin Company.

Autrey, J. (1991). *Love and profit.* New York: William Morrow & Co.

Begley, S. (1994, Nov. 28). Science of the sacred. *Newsweek, 56-59.*

Bellah, R. et al. (1985). *Habits of the heart.* New York: Harper and Row.

Bellah, R. et al. (1991). *The good society.* New York: Alfred Knopf.

Bennett, W. (1994a). *The book of virtues.* New York: Simon and Schuster.

Bennett, W. (1994b). *The index of leading cultural indicators.* New York: Simon and Schuster.

Bennis, W. (1989). *On becoming a leader.* Reading, MA: Addison-Weasley Publishing Co.

Blatt, B. (1981). *In and out of mental retardation.* Baltimore, MD: University Park Press.

Blonston, G. (1992, Sept. 13). The American dream. *Philadelphia Inquirer.* Philadelphia.

Bloom A. (1987). *The closing of the American mind.* New York, NY: Simon and Schuster.

Brown, J. (1991). *Life's little instruction book.* Nashville, TN: Rutledge Hill Press.

Buechner, F. (1993). Journey toward wholeness. *Theology Today,* Vol. II.

Buscaglia, L. (1972). *Love.* New Jersey: Charles B. Shack.

Buscaglia, L. (1978). *Personhood.* New York: Fawcett Columbine.

Buscaglia, L. (1984). *Loving each other.* New York: Fawcett-Columbine.

California Task Force to Promote Self-Esteem and Personal and Social Responsibility. (1990). *Toward a state of esteem.* Sacramento: Author.

Carter, S. (1993). *The culture of disbelief.* New York: Basic Books.

Condeluci, A. (1991). *Interdependence. The route to community.* Delray Beach, FL: St. Lucie Press, Inc.

Covey, S. (1989). *The seven habits of highly effective people.* New York: Simon and Schuster.

Csikszentmihlyi, M. (1990). *Flow: The psychology of optimal experience.* New York: Harper Row.

Dass, R. (1972). *Be here now.* New York, NY: Bell Tower.

Dass, R. (1976). *Grist for the mill.* New York, NY: Anchor Press.

Dass, R., & Gorman, P. (1985). *How can I help?* New York, NY: Alfred Knoff.

Dass, R., & Bush, M. (1991). *Compassion in action.* Bell Tower, New York.

DePree, M. (1989). *Leadership is an art.* New York: Dell Publishing.

de Tocquenville, A. (1848). *Democracy in America.* New York: Harper & Row.

Doubleday Dictionary. (1975). New York: Doubleday and Company.

Editors of Canari Press (1993) *Random acts of kindness.* Berkeley, CA: Conari Press.

Einstein, A. (1956). *Out of my later years.* Secaucus, NJ: The Citadel Press.

Ellis, A. (1975). *A new guide to rational living.* New York: Prentice-Hall.

Erikson, E. (1980). *Identity and the life cycle.* New York: WW Norton.

Etzioni, A. (1993). *The spirit of community.* New York: Crown Publishing.

Freud, S. (1938). *The basic writings of Sigmund Freud.* New York: Modern Library.

Freirc, P. (1989). *Pedegogy of the oppressed.* New York: Continuum Press.

Fromm, E., & Yirau, R. (1968). *The nature of man.* London: MacMillan Co.

Fulghum, R. (1990). *It was on fire when I laid down on it.* New York: Villard Press.

Fulghum, R. (1993). *Maybe (Maybe not).* New York: Villard Press.

Gardner, J. (1991). *Building community.* New York: Community Council.

Garrow, D. (1986). *Bearing the cross.* New York: William Morrow & Co.

Gatto, J. T. (1992). *Dumbing us down.* Philadelphia: New Society Publishers.

Gaylin, W. (1979). *Feelings: Our vital signs.* New York: Harper & Row.

Goffman, E. (1959). *Presentation of self in everyday life.* New York: Anchor Books.

Goffman, E. (1963). *Stigma.* New Jersey: Prentice-Hall.

Greenleaf, R. (1977). *Servant leadership.* New York: Paulist Press.

Hall, E. (1976). *Beyond culture.* New York: Doubleday & Co.

Hampton, H. (1987). *Eyes on the prize.* Boston, MA: Blackside Productions.

Hawson, V. (Ed.) (1974). *Gifts of the lotus.* Wheaton, IL: Theosophical Publishing.

Hughes, R. (1993). *Culture of complaint.* New York: Time Warner.

Hunt, M. (1990). *The compassionate beast.* New York: Doubleday.

Illich, I. (1970). *Deschooling society.* New York: Harper & Row.

Illich, I. (1973). *Tools for conviviality.* New York: Harper & Row.

Illich, I. (1980). *Celebration of awareness.* New York: Doubleday.

Ingram, C. (1990). *In the footsteps of Gandhi: Conversations with spiritual social activists.* New York: Parallax.

James, F. (1993, April 11). The decline and fall of America. *The Pittsburgh Post-Gazette.*

Kantrowitz, B. (1993, August 2). Wild in the streets. *Newsweek.* 40-46.

Kantrowitz, B. et al. (1994, Nov. 28). In search of the sacred. *Newsweek,* 53-54.

Kelsey, M. (1981). *Caring.* New York: Paulist Press.

Kidder, R. (1994). *Shared values for a troubled world.* San Francisco, CA: Josey Bass.

King, M. L. (1989). *The trumpet of conscience.* New York: Harper & Row.

Kubler-Ross, E. (1969). *On death and dying.* New York, NY: MacMillan.

Kohn, A. (1990). *The brighter side of human nature.* New York: Basic Books.

Kohn, A. (1990, Spring). The case against competition. *Noetic Sciences Review.*

Kohn, A. (1986), *No contest.* New York: Basic Books.

Koble, K. (1990). *The cognitive connection.* New York: Addison- Wesley Publishing Co.

Kozol, J. (1985). *Illiterate America.* New York: Doubleday.

Kozol, J. (1987). *Rachael and her children.* New York: Crown Publishers.

Kushner, H. (1982). *When bad things happen to good people.* New York: Schocken Press.

Maslow, A. (1968). *Toward a psychology of being.* New York: Van Nostrand Reinhold.

Maslow, A. (1954). *Motivation and personality.* New York: Harper & Row.

May, R. (1981) *Freedom and destiny.* New York: WW Norton.

Montagu, A., & Matson, F. (1983). *The dehumanization of man.* New York: McGraw Hill.

Morris, D. (1969). *The human zoo.* New York: McGraw Hill.

Morris, D. (1971). *Intimate behavior.* New York: Random House.

Moore, T. (1992). *Care of the soul.* New York: Harper Collins.

Moyer, B. (1987). *A world of ideas.* New York, NY: Doubleday.

Newman, K. (1989). *Falling from grace.* New York: Vintage Books.

Orwell, G. (1945). *Animal farm.*

Pines, A., Aronson, E., & Kafry, D. (1981). *Burn out from tedium to personal growth.* New York: The Free Press.

Roger, J., & McWilliams, P. (1990). *Life 101.* Los Angeles: Prehode Press.

Sagan, C., & Druyan, A. (1992). *Shadows of a forgotten ancestor.* New York: Random House.

Schell, D. W. (1990). *Getting bitter or getting better.* St. Mienrad, IN: Abbey Press.

Siegle, B. (1989). *Love, medicine, and miracles.* New York: Harper and Row.

Senge, P. M. (1990). *The fifth discipline.* New York: Doubleday.

Shapiro, J. (1993). *No pity.* New York: Times Book.

Sher, B., & Gottlieb, A. (1979). *Wishcraft.* New York: Viking Press.

Simon, S. (1990). *Acts of compassion.* New York: Warner Books.

Smedes, L. (1984). *Forgive and forget.* New York: Harper & Row.

Solzhenitsyn, A. (1973). *Gulag Archepeligo.* New York: Harper & Row.

Vanier, J. (1973). *Followers of Jesus.* Toronto: Griffith Press.

Wheatley, M. (1992). *Leadership and the new science.* San Francisco: Barette-Koehler.

Wolfensberger, W. (1987). *The new genocide of handicapped and affected people.* Syracuse, New York: New York Training Institute for Human Service Planning, Leadership and Change Agency.

Wolfensberger, W. (1972). *Normalization.* Toronto: National Institute on Mental Retardation.

Wright, J. E. (1982). *Erickson identity and religion.* New York: Seabury Press.

Yuker, H. (1988). *Attitudes toward persons with disabilities.* New York: Springer Publishers.

Index

A

Acceptance, 13, 21-26, 35, 60, 106, 114, 186-188, 205
Achievement, 172, 199
ADA, 203-204
Age, 9, 59-61, 71-72, 85, 140-142
AIDS, 10, 45, 54-55, 62, 187
Alcoholic, 14
Americans with Disabilities Act, 61, 187, 202
Anti-defamation league, 7

B

Bellah, Robert, 198-199
Blind, 64, 157
Brain-injured, 64

C

Civil rights, 7, 69-70, 107, 184-186, 202, 229
Civil Rights Act, 8, 70
Clinton, Bill, 202
Community, 9-13, 95-96, 114-123, 130-131, 143, 168, 205-215
Compassion, 56, 63, 65, 81-83, 103-104, 167-175, 190, 201, 204, 213-218, 220-225
Consciousness, 15-16, 110, 114, 145, 157, 163, 167-168, 189-193, 200, 204-208, 211-215

D

I

J

K

L

M

S

T

V